NUTRIENTS
A TO Z

D1637967

The hope of humanity lies in the prevention of degenerative and mental diseases, not in the care of their symptoms.

Dr Alexis Carrel

To Debbie

Also from Prion
the companion title

COMPLETE NUTRITION
How to Live in Total Health

Dr Michael Sharon

NUTRIENTS
A TO Z

Dr Michael Sharon, Ph.D

PRION

Published in 1998 in Great Britain by
Prion Books Limited,
32–34 Gordon House Road,
London NW5 1LP

A catalogue record for this book is available from the British
Library.

ISBN 1-85375-261-4

Cover design by Bob Eames
Printed in Great Britain by
Creative Print and Design, Wales

*This book has been designed as a quick reference dictionary
for nutritional information. Its contents are strictly educative
and are not intended to be diagnostic or prescriptive. The
publishers, author and editors do not imply or intend that this
book should in any way replace medical consultation or the
services of a physician.*

PREFACE

Nutritional knowledge is in high demand. 'Back to nature' awareness has become a way of life for many thousands of people and nutritional supplements, organic produce, health foods and rediscovered herbs are the talk of the day. People are taking more responsibility for their own well-being and the result is a greater need for nutritional information conveniently available and easily understood.

This book is intended to serve as a nutritional dictionary, a quick reference book for lay people as well as professionals. It is meant to provide basic information on various nutritional issues, and can easily be used at home or while shopping in the health food store.

We each react differently to foods, and this includes health foods, nutrients and herbs. Sometimes, we even have opposite effects and reactions. This should be remembered when trying to use supplements for the first time: nutrients and herbs must be adapted to the individual. It should also be remembered that the information included in this book is based on average effects that apply to most people, but not necessarily to everybody. Most important of all – do not self-diagnose. In cases of conditions suggestive of symptoms discussed in this book, please consult a natural health care specialist or a holistic doctor for professional advice.

Following the success of its more comprehensive predecessor, *Complete Nutrition*, I hope that this new book will serve to increase public awareness of the exciting connection between nutrition, well-being and longevity. Due to misinformation, many people unknowingly consume harmful foods which act as an enemy. Let us make food our ally. In the words of Hippocrates, 'let us make food our medicine'.

My acknowledgements go to Deborah Ackland MSc, for her continuous advice and support, to my publisher Barry Winkleman, who was the inspiring force behind this publication, and to my dedicated editors Andrew Goodfellow and Mary Warren, who together spared no effort in editing the manuscript. May they all be blessed.

Dr Michael Sharon

HOW TO SOURCE YOUR NUTRIENTS

The various nutrients outlined in the following pages – fruit, vegetables, oils, herbs, vitamins, minerals and supplements – can be found in a wide variety of locations from the obvious to the less obvious. Increasingly, supermarkets and grocers are stocking a wider variety of produce from around the world and many of the foods, herbs and spices that were once thought of as a rarity can be readily located with a minimum of effort. As health becomes more of an issue too, foods with a healing dimension are increasingly available in supermarkets, local stores and grocers.

For more specialist nutrients you may need to take a trip to your local health food store where help and advice is available. Here in addition to nutritious foods and herbs you will find a multitude of vitamins, minerals and nutrients in capsule form and the many compound nutritional formulas that are often tailored toward helping a specific condition. Pharmacies also increasingly serve the health food market with a wide range of vitamins, minerals and supplements. Health food stores obviously vary in size and some of the more specialist nutrients may be available only from larger outlets.

Specialist herbs may again be harder to find, especially fresh herbs. Whereas the health food shop is an increasingly familiar sight on our streets and may offer a range of herbal products, the herbalist is still something of a rarity. At the back of the book is a list of helpful addresses which includes herbalist associations who can offer general advice and herbal suppliers and mail–order companies both in the UK and the US.

Information on sourcing a nutrient is contained within each individual entry. For dosage you should always consult the instructions on the packaging and, for specific conditions, always consult a knowledgeable medical practitioner.

Within the following A to Z, as well as entries on every kind of nutrient, there are also entries on key terms and more general topics within the field of nutrition. They are intended to go some way to helping guide the reader through the vast field of information available on the subject.

Where relevant, within each entry, some of the other key terms or nutrients discussed have been marked in bold to let the reader know that there is a separate entry in the book on that particular subject.

The index at the back of the book complements the main A to Z by covering all the medical and health complaints that are mentioned within these nutritional entries.

A

ACACIA *(Acacia Senegal)*

Also known as gum arabic, it is obtained from the sap of the variety of acacia tree native to North Africa, and has traditionally been used to soothe inflammations of the respiratory, digestive and urinary tracts. Gum arabic is usually dissolved in water to make a mucilage (1–4 teaspoonfuls per cup of water) which can be used to alleviate coughs, sore throats, diarrhoea and dysentery. In addition to its medicinal uses, gum arabic is also used commercially in the making of confectionery, particularly Middle Eastern sweetmeats, and as a thickener (E414) in the preparation and cooking of some foods. Available from larger health food stores, commercial food suppliers and herbalists.

ACID–ALKALINE BALANCE

Although the body has its own natural acid–alkaline balancing mechanisms, an over-indulgence of acidic foods – especially the rich and spicy foods which tend to form the basis of the modern Western diet – can impair this delicate balance. A healthy body needs to be slightly alkaline (pH 7.35–7.45) to counteract these effects. This alkalinity serves as a natural buffer against acid-forming conditions such as stress, lack of exercise, poor eating habits or chronic constipation.

The digestion of acid-forming foods (meat, fish, poultry, eggs, most dairy products, and most grains and pulses) produces acidic residues which need to be eliminated. Excess acidity in body tissues (acidosis) can result in metabolic and respiratory problems and cause many diseases from arthritis to colds and infections. Severe acidosis can occur in diabetes and kidney disease. Excess alkalinity (alkalosis) is quite rare; it can result from taking too many antacid drugs or as a result of frequent vomiting.

Since alkalinity neutralizes acidity, in conditions of mild acidity, the balance can be restored by a diet containing plenty of alkaline foods. Most fruits and vegetables are alkalizing, as are soybeans, lima beans, millet and buckwheat. Milk is neutral. Among the most alkaline-forming foods are figs, carrots, celery and pineapple.

ACIDOPHILUS, LACTOBACILLUS

Intestinal bacteria (flora), which are the 'friendly' bacteria living in the gut, are vital for the proper absorption of nutrients; they also inhibit the growth of the candida albicans yeast (thrush). The Lactobacillus acidophilus bacteria are abundant in yogurts and serve to strengthen the intestinal flora. They can alleviate, and even prevent, a wide range of conditions, including intestinal putrefaction (food decaying in the intestines), vaginal yeast infections, constipation and flatulence. Their main antagonists are antibiotics, which kill all micro-organisms, whether 'friend' or 'foe'. Thus, when on antibiotics, it is very important to replenish the flora by eating plenty of **yoghurt** and by supplementing with acidophilus capsules.

AGAR *(ALSO AGAR-AGAR)*

A gelatinous substance produced from certain species of
Japanese seaweeds, especially the Gelidium variety. Agar is
unaffected by **enzymes** and, since seaweed is rich in minerals
and vitamins, it provides an important source of nutrients. It is
often used as a stabilizing agent (E406) in ice cream and
other foods, and has traditionally been used by the Japanese
as a form of gelatin. As such, agar is superior to the animal-
derived gelatins in that it contains no calories, has a firmer
texture and does not easily melt. It is available from health
food shops as either flakes or bars, and dissolves readily in
boiling water. It is easily digestible, making it particularly
beneficial for sick people and children and, due to its ability
to absorb water and increase in bulk, it is also useful as a
laxative. (See also CARRAGEENAN)

AGRIMONY *(AGRIMONIA EUPATORIA)*

A perennial herb which grows wild in Northern Europe, it
has astringent and anti-inflammatory properties and contains
tannins which can tone the mucous membranes of the gut.
Prepared as a herbal tea or infusion, it can have a very
beneficial effect on the digestive organs – stomach,
intestines, gallbladder and liver – and can also alleviate
inflammation of the intestines caused by food irritants or
infections (enteritis). As an infusion, it can be used as a
gargle for treating mouth infections and is also helpful in
the treatment of diarrhoea. Available from herbalists and
health food stores.

ALCOHOL

Although the consumption of alcoholic beverages has been central to the social rituals of mankind throughout recorded history, nutritionally, alcohol has little to recommend it. As with **wine and beer**, if consumed in moderation, particularly in a social setting, it can add to the pleasure of the occasion and thereby reduce stress. However, it can become addictive and, consumed to excess, alcohol has extremely detrimental effects on the body's metabolism.

The alcohol in beverages is produced by the fermentation of fruit sugars and, when this is metabolized by the body, it produces a harmful chemical called acetaldehyde. It is this that causes the well-known after-effects, or 'hangovers', that so often afflict drinkers. As in the case of refined sugar, alcohol can deplete the body of essential B vitamins, vitamin C, vitamin K, zinc, magnesium and potassium. Even moderate consumption reduces the liver's ability to metabolize glucose and eliminate waste poisons, while higher consumption can result in liver and brain damage, ruptured blood vessels, agglutinated blood, varicose veins, haemorrhoids, thrombosis, damage to the prostate gland and sterility. Alcohol can also increase the possibility of developing age-related diseases such as heart attacks, cataracts and skin wrinkles, and psychological disorders such as anxiety, depression, mental retardation and distorted emotions.

Vitamin B1, niacin, vitamin C and the amino acid cysteine can be helpful in protecting the body from some of the harmful effects of alcohol, and cravings can be alleviated by nutritional supplementation. The Chinese herb **kudzu** as well as the amino acid L-glutamine can be effective in this way and both are available in health food shops. Sometimes, the craving can be due to hypoglycaemia (low blood sugar).

This can be verified by a Glucose Tolerance Test (GTT), and in these cases a suitable diet prescribed by a nutritionist can help.

ALDER *(Alnus Glutinosa)*

A small tree which is found wild throughout the British Isles and Europe. Traditionally, infusions of the shredded bark can relieve constipation and stimulate **bile** secretion, which is necessary for the process of digestion. Decoctions (boiled and simmered teas) can be used to make poultices to ease rheumatic joints, while infusions of the leaves can be used to treat inflammations. Available from larger health food stores, or herbalists.

ALFALFA *(Medicago Sativa)*

A legume, it is a member of the pea family, and is widely grown in Europe, North and South America, Asia and Australia. The seeds and sprouts of the plant are an excellent source of beta carotene and many key nutrients. They are especially rich in minerals (potassium, iron, phosphorus, magnesium, calcium) and vitamins B1, B3, B12, D, C, E and K). The sprouts are widely available in supermarkets and health food shops and are popularly eaten in salads; they can also be used to make alfalfa tea. Alfalfa acts as a tonic, stimulant, appetizer and diuretic, and can assist in the relief of urinary disorders and the alleviation of water retention (oedema).

ALLERGY, FOOD

A food allergy is an abnormal immune system reaction to a substance in food. Normally, when hostile substances enter the blood, the immune system promptly reacts by producing antibodies to engulf and destroy them. In allergic conditions, however, the immune system reacts with the same hostility to certain 'innocent' substances, releasing histamine. This can cause a wide variety of distressing symptoms, from a simple rash to headaches and hypertension.

The causes of allergies are not fully understood by science, although it is known that either the protein parts of foods or dust can trigger the allergies. Some common causes of food allergies are low levels of stomach acid and a shortage of certain pancreatic digestive enzymes. The pancreas secretes enzymes which break down protein into its components, the **amino acids**. A shortage of these enzymes can result in partly digested protein and it is these protein fragments which can induce food allergies in the intestines which produce not only physical, but also mental, symptoms.

Some common food additives, such as benzoic acid (E210) and tartrazine (E102) are known to cause allergic reactions in people with sensitivities, especially in children.

The most common allergenic foods are cow's milk, eggs, chocolate, oranges, wheat, cheese, tomatoes, beef and maize, while among the least allergenic foods are rice, peas and avocados. A craving for a specific food can signal a food allergy and the detection of these allergy-causing foods can be done by the 'pulse test' (see *Complete Nutrition*). A number of nutrients can alleviate or cure these allergies, including **vitamin C** and **quercetin**, both potent antihistamines, **vitamin B6**, **zinc**, **vitamin E** and **calcium**. In fact, some nutritionists believe that allergies may be caused by nutrient deficiencies.

ALMOND

One of the few alkaline nuts, almond is highly respected and valued in traditional Indian medicine (Ayurveda). It can help to relieve phlegm, alleviate coughs and lubricate the intestines. It can also be used for lung conditions and some types of constipation, especially when prepared as a drink by soaking the almonds overnight in water before peeling off the outer brown skin and then blending the nuts with water in a blender. Since almonds are low in two essential **amino acids**, **lysine** and **isoleucine**, as far as their amino acid profile is concerned, they are best complemented for protein utilization by pulses such as beans, peas, chickpeas, lentils, peanuts and soybeans. Almond oil extracts are used mainly for cosmetic purposes. Available from supermarkets and health food stores.

ALOE VERA

A perennial plant which is indigenous to tropical areas of the Far East, southern Africa and the West Indies, it is now cultivated in some of the arid states of the USA, and is also grown in many places as a decorative plant. Nutritionally and medicinally, the plant is useful for the thick juice of its long leaves which has strong anti-fungal and anti-bacterial properties.

The aloe vera juice contains many important vitamins and minerals, as well as beta carotene, enzymes, amino acids and a complex type of carbohydrates called mucopolysaccharides. These are responsible for its many healing actions, which include the soothing of inflammations of the digestive tract and the relief of constipation, flatulence and the symptoms of irritable bowel syndrome (IBS). The gelatinous juice of the fresh leaves can also be used externally. It is reputed to heal wounds and can also be rubbed on the skin to alleviate sunburns, wrinkles, skin irritations and minor cuts. Infusions are good for bathing wounds and eyes. The juice has a somewhat repellent taste and, when taken internally, it is usually blended with fruit juice to make it more palatable. Pure American aloe vera juice is now readily available in most health foods shops.

ALUMINIUM

Everyday sources of this toxic element are processed cheeses, baking soda, antacid tablets, table salt and antiper-spirants (E173). It can also be ingested through the use of aluminium cookware and utensils. Aluminium disturbs the calcium–phosphorus balance and causes the loss of vitamin B1 and excesses of aluminium salts, which can accumulate in the brain, are implicated in the loss of memory, presenile dementia and Alzheimer's disease. Vitamin C is recommended to counteract the build up of these salts in the body, as well as **garlic**, **seaweeds** and **wheat grass**.

AMARANTH (*AMARANTHUS HYPOCHONDRIACUSA*)

The grain is also known as Inca wheat and was the main staple of the Aztec diet due to its high protein content. It is now cultivated commercially in the American Midwest and incorporated into some breakfast cereals. The crimson flowers have an astringent property and infusions of these can be effective in the treatment of diarrhoea and dysentery; they can also be used to reduce excessive menstrual bleeding. Amaranth is normally sold as a prepared cereal, but the flowers may also be obtainable from some herbalists.

AMINO ACIDS

Amino acids are the building blocks of proteins. They are made up of carbon, hydrogen, oxygen, sulphur and iron, and to create the many forms of proteins in the body, the amino acids link together to form the various chain structures (peptides) that give each kind of protein – whether in bone, hair or nails, etc. – its specific characteristics. The formation of these various proteins is governed by other proteins, the nucleic acids DNA and RNA, often described as genetic 'blueprints'. DNA contains the master code and RNA conveys its message to the cells where the different kinds of protein are formed. Protein synthesis is vitally important for sustaining life as cells are constantly being broken down and must be recreated.

Of the 24 known amino acids that make up the thousands of differing protein combinations, eight of these – leucine, isoleucine, valine, methionine, threonine, lysine, phenylalanine and tryptophan – are known as the 'essential amino acids' as all eight must be present simultaneously in the diet, and in the right proportions, in order to form what is termed 'complete protein'. None of these can be synthesized by the human body for itself and must be acquired from food. If even one is absent, or in a disproportionately low ratio to the others, then protein synthesis is halted or reduced. In this case, what is formed is termed 'incomplete protein'. This can happen in the diets of strict vegetarians (vegans) subsisting on 'incomplete' vegetable protein, as it is the animal foods such as meat, fish, eggs and dairy produce which contain all the 'essentials' and form 'complete protein'. Individual free amino acids have been found to have specific beneficial effects, such as burning off fat, treating baldness, building muscle or relieving stress and, as such, they can be used as nutritional supplements. Some amino acids such as arginine, which are not adequately produced in many people, are considered 'semi–essential'.

ANGELICA *(ANGELICA ARCHANGELICA)*

Angelica is a large aromatic plant native to Northern Europe and Asia, which can be either biennial or perennial, and is found in damp places such as river banks. It is also cultivated. For nutritional and medicinal purposes, the useful parts of the plant are its roots and seeds.

Angelica tea, which can be produced from both the roots and the seeds, will aid digestion, relieve flatulence and stimulate appetite. It is useful for a number of digestive problems, including ulcers, vomiting and colic. Applied externally, as a lotion, Angelica can help relieve rheumatic pain and gout. A decoction of the root can be applied to the skin to treat scabies or itching.

An infusion can be made by adding half a cup of boiling water to one teaspoon of crushed seeds and steeping; a decoction can be made by boiling one teaspoon crushed root in 3/4 cup of water, and then steeping for five minutes.

For convenience, Angelica is sold as a liquid extract by some herbalists and the larger health food stores. This can be taken in a dosage of 10 to 30 drops in liquid, three times daily.

Caution: Angelica must not be taken by diabetics as it

tends to elevate blood sugar level.

ANISE, ANISEED *(PIMPINELLA ANISUM)*

Anise is an aromatic plant that is native to the
Mediterranean regions, but is also cultivated. Its sweet seeds
are used in Mediterranean cooking, mainly for flavouring.
As an infusion, anise helps digestion, relieves flatulence,
improves appetite and alleviates cramps, nausea and colic in
children.

As a tisane, anise can be used to stimulate milk production in nursing mothers and an infusion of the seeds is
reputed to bring on delayed menstruation. A tisane is made
by boiling half a teaspoon crushed seed in half a pint water
and straining it. An infusion is made with one teaspoon
crushed seed boiled with a cup of water and allowed to
steep for ten minutes.

Anise is also known to promote energy circulation and
increase the metabolic rate, which is valuable in any weight-
loss programme. Available from larger health food stores and
herbalists.

ANTACIDS

Antacid drugs bring only temporary relief, not a permanent
cure, and, unless prescribed, anyone using antacids should
realize that the symptoms of too much acid in the stomach
are similar to those of having too little. In the latter case,
therefore, taking antacids will only serve to exacerbate the
problem. In addition, some antacids contain **aluminium**, a
toxic element which can build up in the body and give rise
to an array of disorders.

Heartburn resulting from low acidity in the stomach can be relieved with betaine HCl tablets. In fact, since stomach secretions are known to diminish with age, some authorities recommend that anyone over 40 should use a HCl supplement with each main meal.

In some cases, digestive enzymes such as **pancreatin tablets** can help, but correct **food combinations** are considered to be the simplest and most effective way of preventing stomach over-acidity, heartburn and dyspepsia.

For quick relief, it is best taking 2–3 **dolomite** tablets with each meal. In the author's experience, a glass of cold milk or a few raw almonds can be very effective in cases of heartburn. Another simple way to avoid heartburn is to drink fluids before meals, rather than after, as this dilutes gastric juices.

ANTIBIOTICS

Once thought to eradicate all infectious diseases, the use of antibiotics is beginning to decline. While sensitivities to the drugs are on the increase, their actual effectiveness in treatments has decreased. Several strains of bacteria have developed immunity and resist antibiotic treatments. It is now estimated that 20 per cent of infections contracted in hospitals fail to respond to antibiotic treatment, and in the US alone more than 100,000 people die each year from such infections.

Originally, antibiotics were very powerful and their use in emergencies saved many lives, but unfortunately doctors developed a tendency to prescribe antibiotics indiscriminately and eventually, as a result of overuse, many bacteria developed resistance to the drugs and it became necessary to prescribe higher and higher doses. In time, a vicious cycle was formed as the higher doses created stronger side-effects.

Since antibiotics are unable to distinguish between micro-organisms, they kill the 'friendly' intestinal bacteria (flora) needed for food absorption along with the pathogenic bacteria. One of the results of this has been a proliferation of vaginal yeast infections in women who have been pre-scribed tetracyclines. Antibiotics can also neutralize the effects of the contraceptive pill. As a result, doctors are now reserving the use of antibiotics as a last resort and there is a growing tendency to prepare patients for surgery by fortifying their immune system over a period of time with balanced, well-supplemented diets.

ANTIDEPRESSANTS, NUTRITIONAL

Nutritional treatment of depression, stress and anxiety can include two of the **amino acids**: DLPA (DL-phenylalanine), which increases levels of noradrenaline and dopamine in the brain, and GABA (gamma-aminobutyric acid), which is gaining popularity for its anti-anxiety effects. The latter is derived in the body from glutamic acid and acts as an inhibitory neurotransmitter. That is, it slows down the fran-tic activity of the nerve cells in the brain's lymbic system, which is the body's emotional alarm bell.

Calcium is a well-known calming mineral which can even alleviate insomnia if taken at bedtime at doses of 500 mg. Helpful vitamins for treating stress and depression are Vitamin C and the B vitamins, expecially B1, niacin and pantothenic acid, while beneficial herbs include **hawthorn**, **kava kava**, **linden**, **St John's wort** and **valerian**.

Among the foods that can acerbate depression and anxiety and should be avoided are white sugar, white flour, caffeine and a high-fat diet. Similarly, alcohol consumption and smoking should be reduced or cut out completely.

ANTIOXIDANTS

Antioxidants are substances that neutralize **free radicals**. These are atoms or molecules that are formed during food metabolism, or by pollutants, smoking and radiation, and are electronically unbalanced. In stable molecules, electrons come in pairs, but free radicals have unpaired electrons – either one is missing or there is an extra one – and to restabilize themselves they grab an electron from another molecule. In this way, another free radical is created and a vicious chain reaction is begun or continued.

Free radicals, unless or until they are neutralized, damage various body cells. For instance, they can distort the DNA genetic blueprint, thus causing many of the degenerative diseases of ageing, such as heart disease, cancer and strokes; they also attack blood vessels producing blood clots and atherosclerosis, and they can damage brain cells, creating memory loss and senility.

The antioxidants serve as free radical scavengers, neutralizing and defending the body from their oxidative damage. The body protects itself with various antioxidant enzymes, such as superoxide dismutase (SOD) and catalase or glutathione peroxide. Free radicals are also neutralized by antioxidant nutrients such as the vitamins A, C, E, B1, B5, B6, niacin and PABA, the amino acid cysteine (found in eggs), minerals zinc and selenium, catechols (found in bananas and potatoes), phenolics (found in grapes and other fruits), quercetin (found in onion and garlic), rutin (found in buckwheat) and hesperidin (found in citrus rind). Other foods high in natural antioxidants include wheat grass, berries and dark green vegetables.

Commercially, chemical antioxidants such as BHA and BHT are used in processed foods to protect them from spoilage and to prevent colour change from oxidation. BHA (butylated hydroxyanisole), which is widely used as a preservative (E320) in many foods, can be harmful to the kidneys, while BHT (butylated hydroxytoluene), its chemical cousin (E321), can cause even more damage to the kidneys.

APPETITE

For anyone wishing to reduce weight, or needing to curb or control their appetite for other reasons, the following nutrients can be helpful if included in the diet: avocados, bran and fibrous foods, celery stalks, guar gum, hydroxycitric acid (HCA) as in Citrimax tablets, together with the amino acid L-phenylalanine, and also freshly squeezed lemon juice.

For those needing to stimulate their appetite, the following foods are recommended: **alfalfa** sprouts, **apples**, **carrot** juice, **cayenne pepper**, **celery** leaves, chicken, **cider vinegar**, **corn**, **grapefruit**, liver, **mushrooms**, **oranges**, strawberries and **tomatoes**. In addition, herbs such as **agrimony**, **anise** and **camomile**, together with the **vitamin B complex**, **zinc** and **brewer's yeast** are also useful additions to the diet.

APPLES

Apples are a highly nutritious and cleansing fruit, as well as a good source of vitamins A and B1; they are also rich in a number of minerals including potassium, calcium, phosphorus, sodium and the trace elements. In addition, they contain malic and tartaric acids, which inhibit gastric fermentation and bacteria proliferation in the digestive tract.

The fruit are rich in pectin, which has numerous uses: it can help reduce high cholesterol levels and remove toxic metals such as lead and mercury from the body; it is very beneficial for intestinal problems and it binds radioactive residues and excretes them from the body. It is also used as a stabilizer (E440b) in the commercial production of foods such as jams and preserves.

Apples can help cleanse the lungs from phlegm and protect them from smoking; they also boost immunity and stimulate the appetite. In addition, apple juice is very cleansing for the liver and gall bladder.

APRICOTS

Originating in China, apricots are a popular seasonal fruit which ripen in June and July. Ripe apricots are an excellent source of **vitamin A** and **potassium**. A serving of 100 g contains over 80 g of vitamin A. Apricots are recommended eating in cases of lung conditions. They are also high in **copper** and **cobalt** and can therefore be beneficial in the treatment of anaemia. In addition, they contain substantial amount of **calcium**, **silicon**, **phosphorus** and **vitamin C**.

Caution: Apricots should be used cautiously during pregnancy and avoided in cases of diarrhoea.

ARACHIDONIC ACID *(AA)*

It is one of the essential fatty acids, which have numerous duties, and causes the production of prostaglandins (PG) of the type PGE2. These are hormone-like compounds which stimulate and control many bodily functions. PGE2 accelerates blood clotting and increases water retention, but excesses of it, which arise primarily from consumption of animal products, can cause pain and inflammations. AA also releases leukotrienes; these are substances which can help to heal wounds and injuries but, in excess, will stimulate such conditions as breast lumps and arthritis, especially rheumatoid arthritis, asthma, psoriasis and lupus erythematosus. **Aspirin** and steroid drugs inhibit the synthesis of PGE2 and can therefore reduce blood clotting, pain and fever. Indeed, aspirin is now widely used to protect vulnerable people from heart attacks. However, as it also inhibits PGE1, which counteracts the action of PGE2, a better choice is to increase the level of PGE1, which has a natural anti–inflammatory action. This can be done by taking evening primrose oil and excluding animal foods (except for some fish).

ARGININE *(L-ARGININE)*

Arginine is a semi–essential amino acid which, with its derivative ornithine, stimulates the secretion by the pituitary gland of growth hormone in the brain. This is essential not only for children's growth, but also, since it promotes repair of worn tissues and helps to heal wounds, in adults too. In addition, it stimulates the growth of T-lymphocytes – immune cells that identify, engulf and destroy invading bacteria and carcinogenic chemicals. In this respect, arginine – which is abundant in home-made chicken soup – can be extremely useful in the treatment of autoimmune diseases such as arthritis and multiple sclerosis. Arginine and ornithine have also been reported to stimulate weight loss and increase sperm count and motility.

Arginine is usually taken in doses of 2 g on an empty stomach, preferably at bedtime – growth hormone is released naturally at night-time, when peak secretions are reached about 90 minutes after falling asleep. Arginine can also be taken one hour before a strenuous exercise. Ornithine should be taken at half the doses of arginine.

Caution: Arginine and ornithine should not be used by growing children or pregnant and lactating women. Arginine is contra-indicated in herpes.

ARNICA (ARNICA MONTANA)

A perennial plant, which is also known as mountain tobacco, it grows in the mountainous regions of Europe, Siberia, northern Asia and the western United States and Canada. For centuries, it has been widely used as a healing herb, especially for bruising and trauma in cases of accident or injury. However, it should never be used on broken skin or open wounds.

An infusion prepared from the root will stimulate perspiration and help to reduce temperature in a feverish cold; it can also be used to soothe inflamed mucous membranes and nasal passages and act as a diuretic and general stimulant. Infusions can also be applied externally as a hair tonic. Available from larger health food stores and herbalists.

AROMATHERAPY

This is an ancient art which uses aromatic plant essences which, although they are not 'oily' in texture, are known as essential oils. These can be extracted from the flowers, leaves, stems, fruits, seeds and/or roots of the plants and their effects are many and varied. As inhalations or applied to the skin, these essential oils can be used to relieve physical conditions, restore mental and physical balance and create a feeling of well-being.

Aromatic herbs have been used for thousands of years for both healing and cosmetic purposes. For instance, ancient Ayurvedic texts include aromatic essences in many of their treatments, but modern aromatherapy was rediscovered in the 1920s by René-Maurice Gattefossé, a French chemist, who studied the therapeutic effects of essential oils after accidentally discovering the beneficial effects of lavender oil in the treatment of burns.

More recently, with the resurgence of interest in natural living and complementary medicines, aromatherapy too has become increasingly popular. Around three thousand essential oils are used by trained aromatherapists, most of whom use a holistic approach, i.e. they do not treat merely the symptom, but consider the complete physical and emotional state as an entity. An essential oil may contain many different compounds, all working together to provide benefit. Many aromatherapy blends are available which are carefully balanced to produce specific effects such as relaxation, sensuality, clarity and inspiration. For example, a sensual blend can be made from ylang ylang, lavender and sandalwood, while premenstrual tension can be eased with a blend of clary sage and geranium. Essential oils are quickly absorbed, and inhalation is very effective for delivering the active ingredients to the bloodstream. Many essential oils are also very effective as antimicrobial and antifungal agents.

ARTICHOKE *(CYNARA SCOLYMUS)*

A large, thistle-like perennial plant, which originated in the Mediterranean region, it produces edible flower buds and is sometimes known as globe artichoke. It is now widely cultivated in temperate climates, including in the US where the plant is grown commercially, chiefly in California.

The flower heads are commonly eaten as vegetables, but extracts of the leaves and roots were once used to treat arteriosclerosis, jaundice and post-operative anaemia. Artichokes provide a number of vitamins and minerals; they can also stimulate **bile** evacuation and act as a diuretic. In some cultures the artichoke is considered to be an aphrodisiac.

ASCORBIC ACID SEE VITAMIN C

ASPARAGINE

This is a non-essential amino acid which, with glutamic acid, is most commonly found in the brain. It is thought to regulate brain and nerve metabolism, and is used in the treatment of mental and emotional disorders. Available from health food stores.

ASPARAGUS

A nutritious green vegetable, it is a perennial which originated in the Mediterranean region and in Africa. It grows
best in moderate climates and the young shoots, which are
mainly used in cooking, are a rich source of vitamins and
minerals. It is especially rich in vitamin E and two ounces
can provide a good daily dose. Asparagus contains
asparagine, an amino acid, which provides calming properties. The plant is also a diuretic and can aid the elimination
of water through urination, a special boon in cases of water
retention (oedema). Asparagus can be used to treat many
kidney conditions, but it should not be used in cases of
inflammations. It is also helpful in cleansing cholesterol from
arteries and hence is useful in treating vascular problems
such as hypertension and arteriosclerosis.

Caution: In excessive amounts, asparagus can irritate the
kidneys.

ASPARTIC ACID

A non-essential amino acid, it has chelating effects – that is,
it can bind toxic elements such as lead and mercury and
assist in their excretion from the body. Aspartic acid, with
phenylalanine, produces the popular artificial sweetener
Aspartame, which is 160 times sweeter than sugar and is
used mainly in diet soft drinks and sweetening tablets.

ASPIRIN

Aspirin is a non-steroidal anti-inflammatory drug which is
readily obtainable over-the-counter and has become widely

used as an inexpensive form of painkiller. It is commonly used to treat the aches and pains of conditions such as migraines and arthritis. However, aspirin is not a cure; it can only mitigate or alleviate pain and, in spite of its popularity and being freely available, it is not totally harmless. Not only does it deplete the body's supply of vitamin C, large or frequent dosing with aspirin can irritate the stomach and cause stomach haemorrhages and ulcers.

In recent years, aspirin has been widely prescribed in the treatment of arthritis and to protect from heart disease, as it is known to block the production of PGE2, a prostaglandin. This is a hormone-like compound and excesses of it can increase blood–clotting and contribute to heart attack. However, aspirin also inhibits PGE1 and PGE3, which are beneficial prostaglandins that counteract the effects of PGE2. A preferable choice of treatment, therefore, is to increase the body's levels of PGE1 by using supplements such as evening primrose oil and, at the same time, reducing the intake of animal foods.

ASTRAGALUS (Astragalus Mambranaceus)

A traditional Chinese herb, its root was found to increase resistance to disease by fortifying the immune system. For example, it increases the body's secretion of interferon, which fights viruses. According to Chinese studies, astragalus reduces proneness to colds and their duration. Astragalus is indicated, together with echinacea and ginseng, for use in the degenerative diseases of ageing such as heart disease, cancer and arthritis. Since it is a diuretic, astragalus can be useful to reduce water retention (oedema). During the past decade, astragalus has been 'discovered' by Western science, and is increasingly being incorporated into nutritional formulas sold in health food shops.

AUBERGINE

A tropical plant, which is also known as the eggplant, its non-starchy fruit combine well with other foods and provide a versatile ingredient in casseroles, dips and salads. It is high in fibre, low in fat and contains an array of nutrients, such as vitamins A and C, niacin and folic acid, and the minerals iron, calcium, magnesium and potassium. It is also rich in antioxidant bioflavonoids which can provide protection from stomach cancer. In addition, its mucilaginous fibre can help to lower cholesterol levels, while its high potassium content is useful in the prevention of water retention.

Aubergine is reputed to reduce bleeding and has traditionally been used for the treatment of piles, and bleeding in general. It is an astringent food and is useful in the treatment of diarrhoea. It is also very suitable for inclusion in weight loss programmes as one cup of cooked cubes contains only 27 calories, 3 mg of sodium and a trace of fat, but, due to its high fibre content, it provides a feeling of fullness. It is best bought fresh when it is firm, weighty, and free of scars and cuts.

AVOCADO

Native to Mexico, Guatemala, Jamaica, and Cuba, the avocado is now grown in many of the tropical and subtropical regions of the world, particularly in the fruit-growing regions of Florida and California. Rich in vitamins, minerals, and oil, it provides an excellent source of nutritious protein and is often recommended for nursing mothers. It is a good internal lubricator and can be used as a natural remedy for ulcers. It is also known to beautify the skin.

Avocado is a fruit high in **lecithin**, which is a brain food, and most of its calorific value (80 per cent) comes from easily digested fat, mainly monounsaturated fatty acids. It is very beneficial to people with low blood sugar (hypo-glycaemia) as it contains manoheptulose, a special type of sugar which depresses secretion of insulin; thus, in contrast to refined white sugar, it actually prevents low blood sugar. For this reason, avocados can be a valuable contribution to weight loss programmes as they help to satisfy hunger for long periods of time. They are also a useful ingredient for any food-combining diet as they will combine well with both proteins and starches.

B

BABIES, FOOD

It is most important to breast feed for the first six months at least, if at all possible. As the mother's early milk (colostrum) is rich in antibodies and lymphocytes, which boost the immunity of the child to diseases, later breast feeding largely determines the baby's health; not only in the first few months, but for many years to come, and saves needless miseries such as ear infections, colics and allergies. Research has shown that the substitution of cow's milk in the early months can be correlated with later obesity and heart disease. It would seem that the high cholesterol level in a mother's milk – as opposed to low cholesterol in cow's milk – serves in fact to establish lower cholesterol levels in later years. Recent studies have also indicated that when cow's milk is introduced in early infancy, before four months of age, this may trigger the autoimmune process and increase the risk of diabetes developing in later years.

From the age of six months, mashed vegetables and other foods should be introduced gradually, while at the same time decreasing the consumption of milk. Then, when the first molar appears – usually at about 18 months – this is a sign that the pancreatic enzymes in the intestines are ready to synthesize more solid foods. Of course, this is only a general timetable and every baby is different: some can be weaned at a very early age while others will refuse weaning even after the first birthday. When mother's milk is not available it is advisable to use either the milk from another mother (a wet nurse) or goat milk, or a combination of both. Babies born to vegan mothers are known to thrive on almond milk or soya milk.

BACTERIA, INTESTINAL see PROBIOTICS

BAKING SODA, BAKING POWDER

Baking soda or baking powder, which are commonly used to leaven bread, deplete two of the B vitamins, thiamine and folic acid, and neutralize vitamin C. They also contain **aluminium salts**, which can accumulate in the brain and damage brain cells, causing memory loss and pre senile dementia. One way to avoid this is by using the sourdough leavening process. In this method, the starter is made from just flour and water which is allowed to stand for three days, by which time live airborne yeast will have turned the mix sour.

Baking soda (sodium bicarbonate) provides a very useful dentrifice as it neutralizes acidic plaque and prevents gum infections. It can also eliminate bacteria that causes tooth decay. A simple cure for athlete's foot is to dust the affected area with baking soda.

Caution: Baking soda should not be used as an antacid for stomach over-acidity or heartburn by people on low-sodium diets.

BALM, LEMON BALM *(MELISSA OFFICINALIS)*

A perennial plant, originally native to the eastern
Mediterranean, it can now be found growing wild throughout most of Europe, but is mainly cultivated as a culinary
herb for its lemon-scented leaves. An infusion of the leaves
can be used to dull pain, ease toothache, and relieve flatulence,
cramps, indigestion and colic. Since it increases perspiration, it
is useful in treating colds by reducing feverishness.
Traditionally, it has been used to treat nervousness, depression and insomnia, and it is also claimed to stimulate the
onset of menstruation and relieve period pains. The leaves
can be used to prepare a pleasant, aromatic tea which has
soothing and relaxing properties. Available from larger
health food stores and herbalists.

BANANA

An aromatic fruit, which originated in Asia, it is now grown
in the hot, damp climates of the tropic regions of both the
eastern and western hemispheres. Bananas are rich in potassium and are used to treat hypertension, and detoxify the
body. Their principal aroma is amyl acetate and they contain
large amounts of tryptophan, an amino acid which is converted to serotonin, an inhibiting brain neurotransmitter
that reduces nerve activity. Hence, they are a calming food,
especially (when taken with milk) before bedtime.

   Bananas can serve as a good internal lubricator for the
intestines as they moisten dryness and, although they are
commonly given to children, they are also a very suitable
food for elderly people who tend to suffer from hypertension, weak digestion and general weakness. Bananas are
astringent before fully ripened, which makes them useful in

the treatment of diarrhoea and haemorrhoids. When fully ripe, bananas can be beneficial in the treatment of constipation and ulcers.

BARBERRY *(BERBERIS VULGARIS)*

The common barberry is a deciduous shrub which grows wild throughout Europe and the eastern United States. Both its roots and berries can be used in infusions. An infusion of the root promotes the secretion of bile and is therefore beneficial in liver disorders. It also tends to dilate blood vessels and so can help to lower blood pressure. The bark of the root has a laxative effect. Decoctions of either the root or berries make a good mouthwash or gargle for mouth and throat irritations. Available from herbalists.

Caution: Neither high nor low blood pressure should be treated with barberry.

BARLEY

Probably one of the first cultivated cereals, barley is grown in almost all the temperate regions of Europe and North America. It is a nutritious and easily digested cereal, providing a good source of fibre, iron, calcium and protein. It is known to strengthen the stomach and intestines and soothe inflamed membranes, and is believed to help reduce tumours and oedema. It can be used in the alleviation of painful urination and as a mild laxative. Sprouted barley is even more nutritious and can help indigestion and abdominal bloating. It is also a strong blood purifier.

Barley grass, which can be grown at home, is richer in chlorophyll, vitamin A and enzymes, making it easier to digest. It also contains the antioxidant enzyme **SOD** and mucopolysaccharides which give it anti-inflammatory properties. Barley grass has a high protein content of 20 per cent, about the same as that of meat.

Barley malt is a sweetener prepared from sprouted barley. During sprouting, starch is converted to maltose, which does not harm teeth as sugar does and is therefore a much safer and more nutritious sweetener. Ground roasted barley is frequently used as an ingredient in several brands of coffee substitutes and is recommended as a relief for fatigue. Available in health food shops.

BASIL *(Ocimum Basilicum)*

An annual with a pungent aroma, the plant is native to India but has been grown throughout the Mediterranean regions for thousands of years. It is now cultivated throughout southern and western Europe as an aromatic culinary herb. The leaves have appetite-stimulating properties and are generally used as a culinary flavouring. Infusions of the leaves can be used to relieve flatulence, fermentation, stomach cramps and constipation and the plant is also said to relieve nausea. Available from supermarkets.

BAY LEAVES SEE LAUREL

BEANS SEE LEGUMES

BEARBERRY (ARCTOSTAPHYLOS UVA-URSI)

Bearberry, also called uva ursi, is an evergreen shrub of the Ericaceae family. It has small bitter leaves and produces juicy but insipid berries. The leaves contain tannins, which are astringents, and glycosides, which are excellent antiseptics and anti-bacterial. Until the advent of antibiotics, bearberry was used as a urinary tract antiseptic. The astringent properties of the leaves can also be utilized in an infusion which can help to alleviate diarrhoea and bleeding. Bearberry also has diuretic properties and can be used to reduce uric acid levels, for the relief of pain caused by kidney stones and gravel, and for the alleviation of the symptoms of chronic cystitis. Available from larger health food stores and herbalists.

Caution: Excessive use of bearberry can cause stomach pain.

BEE POLLEN

Pollen is the yellowish dust produced by the anthers of male flowers. It is transferred by bees to the ovaries of the female flowers resulting in their fertilization and the development of fruit or seeds. Specific types of pollen are also collected by bees for storage in their hives as food for the young bees.

The composition of bee pollen varies according to the type of flower it has come from but, whatever its source, it is one the most nourishing foods available to mankind. On average, it contains 30 per cent amino acids (protein), 50 per cent carbohydrates, 14 per cent polyunsaturated fatty acids, a large concentration of minerals and trace elements, many of the A, C, D, E and B- complex vitamins and bioflavonoids. The protein is complete and rates higher than meat in essential amino acids. Nutritionally, it is so perfectly balanced that, in itself, it represents a complete survival food.

Bee pollen has been extensively studied for its beneficial effects. It has been given to athletes as it has been found to improve energy and endurance; in the Republic of Georgia, the consumption of bee pollen has been correlated with longevity. Bee pollen has also been found to prevent colds and flu, help the immune system to fight virus infections, relieve fatigue, improve appetite, increase sexual potency and fertility, alleviate painful menstruation, reduce the hot flushes of menopause for women and alleviate enlarged prostate in men.

Bee pollen is considerably less allergenic than wind-borne pollens. It should be taken regularly for at least one month: up to 20 grams a day provides a normal supplement, while 40 grams constitutes a therapeutic dosage. Available from larger health food stores.

BEER SEE WINE & BEER

BEET *(BETA VULGARIS)*

Table beet is a vegetable that originally grew wild in the Mediterranean regions. It is rich in iron and also contains vitamins B1, B2, C, and the minerals potassium, manganese, phosphorus and silicon. Although, normally, it is the root part of the plant that is eaten, in fact its leaves are a good source of beta carotene. Beet has a number of useful medicinal properties. For instance, it can be used for purifying the blood, improving circulation, promoting menstruation and stimulating the bowels. Beet can also be helpful for the treatment of liver problems as well as constipation. Some healers recommend beet for intestinal cleansing from parasites. In addition, it can help calm nervousness and is of benefit in vascular congestions. Beet can also help to overcome a sweet tooth. Available from supermarkets and grocers.

Caution: Green beets are rich in oxalic acid and, if eaten in excess, they can interfere with calcium metabolism and promote the formation of calcium-oxalate kidney stones.

BELLADONA (ATROPA BELLADONA)

Commonly known as deadly nightshade, this poisonous plant grows wild throughout Europe and many Asian countries. It contains several alkaloids, including atropine, which relieves asthma, hyoscyiamine, which induces sleep and can cause paralysis, belladonine, which is a narcotic and pain killer, and scopolamine, another painkiller which reduces high blood pressure and produces twilight sleep.

Caution: The narcotic action of belladona affects the central nervous system and can cause paralysis. It is available on prescription in tinctures and extracts and it should only be used under medical supervision.

BENZOIC ACID

A commonly used food preservative (E210) in many processed foods, it is known to cause allergies in sensitive people. Children are especially vulnerable and allergic reactions can include hyperactivity, abdominal pains, diarrhoea, asthma and rashes. Saccharin is a derivative of benzoic acid.

BETA CAROTENE

Beta carotene is a vitamin A precursor (also called pro–vitamin A) and one of the many plant pigments known collectively as **carotenoids**. It is the most prevalent carotenoid in plants. These plant pigments are potent antioxidants, protecting the plants from destruction by the free radicals generated by dangerous sun rays and without these protective carotenoids, the plants would quickly shrivel. People can acquire the same protection from **antioxidants** by eating foods high in beta carotene, such as carrots, sweet potatoes, cantaloupe, pumpkin and green leafy vegetables. The micro-algae **spirulina** and dunaliella are among the highest sources of beta carotene.

Although beta carotene is converted to vitamin A in the body, it has additional biological properties of its own. It is a stronger antioxidant than vitamin A and studies have shown that it protects the body from several types of cancer, especially lung cancer. Beta carotene also acts as a filter, protecting eye lens from cataract. In addition, it boosts the immune system and stimulates the T-cells, providing a strong protection to the thymus gland.

BETAINE HCL

This is a stomach acid supplement available at health food shops for people with low gastric secretion. A betaine HCl tablet taken after a meal can improve food tolerance and digestion and its use can also help conditions resulting from low stomach acid, such as heartburn. Since low stomach acid (HCl) is known to cause allergies, betaine HCl can also help reduce various allergy symptoms. Gastric secretions are known to be reduced with age and Dr Alan Nittler, author of *A New Breed of Doctor*, recommends that everyone over the age of 40 should take betaine HCl tablets as a matter of course.

BILBERRY *(VACCINIUM MYRTILLUS)*

Also known as whortleberry, this small perennial plant grows wild in the poor soil of sandy areas and moors and both its berries, which are black, and its leaves can be used for medicinal purposes. Bilberry is rich in flavonoids, particularly proanthocyanidins and anthocyanidins, both of which are powerful antioxidants and have an anti-inflammatory effect, strengthening capillaries and collagen. Bilberry extracts, which are rich in anthocyanidin compounds, are now increasingly used to treat eye conditions such as near-sightedness, and to improve night vision and reverse diabetic retinopathy. An infusion of the leaves is antiseptic and can be used to treat diarrhoea and dysentery; it can also act as a diuretic. Capsules and formulas for improving eyesight are available from larger health food stores.

BILE

A thick fluid secreted by the liver, bile is produced from cholesterol through the action of an enzyme and with the help of vitamin C. It is used by the duodenum to emulsify fats and assist with the absorption of fatty acids. Excess bile is stored in the gall bladder, where it is discharged into the duodenum as it is needed.

A high level of vitamin C in the diet helps to promote bile production, which, in turn, assists in the reduction of cholesterol levels. At the same time, dietary improvement can help to increase the production of bile since, when a diet is low in protein, or high in sugar, little bile is produced. As a result of this, fats are poorly dissolved in the digestive tract and parts of the undissolved fats will then combine with calcium and iron from food to form insoluble soaps. These can be harmful in two respects: they can prevent absorption of calcium and iron, causing deficiencies, and can also harden the stools, causing constipation. A fat-free diet is also undesirable because it does not stimulate bile flow and, as a result of this, sediments may form which can promote the development of gallstones.

BIOAVAILABILITY

This term specifies to what extent various micronutrients in food are absorbed and become available to their target tissues or organs after eating. In other words, it is not a matter of what is consumed, but what the body is able to absorb and assimilate from the foods ingested. There are a variety of factors that can influence bioavailability, such as ageing, food processing, reduced digestive secretions, shortage of enzymes in the body, and nutrient interaction – in which some nutrients inhibit or increase absorption of other nutrients.

BIOFLAVONOIDS *(Vitamin P)*

Bioflavonoids are complex compounds closely associated with vitamin C and found in a wide range of plants, particularly the citrus fruits. All the bioflavonoids enhance the effectiveness of vitamin C, and are recognized as potent antioxidants. Together with vitamin C, they strengthen the capillaries and help prevent excessive menstrual bleeding. They are also anti-viral and anti-inflammatory, protect from free radicals and inhibit histamine release. Bioflavonoids are therefore indicated in inflammatory and allergic conditions.

As a group, several hundred flavonoids have been identified in fruits, vegetables, nuts, seeds, leaves and flowers. Onions and garlic provide rich sources of **quercetin**, a bioflavonoid with potent anti-carcinogenic activity, which has been shown to inhibit the growth of several types of cancer cells, including breast cancer, ovarian cancer and leukaemia. Quercetin has also been found to be effective in healing wounds, preventing diabetic cataracts and in treating oral herpes.

Cherries, hawthorn berries, bilberries and other berries are rich in anthocyanidins and proanthocyanidins, the flavonoids that give berries their dark reddish-blue colour and which are powerful antioxidants, preventing free radical damage and helping to maintain healthy collagen and capillaries. Buckwheat is rich in the bioflavonoid **rutin** which is a well-known treatment for piles, varicose veins and hypertension. Hesperidin, the predominant flavonoid in citrus fruits is chemically similar to rutin. Since bioflavonoids strengthen the capillaries, they can assist in the treatment of duodenal ulcers and retinal haemorrhages.

BIOTIN

A water-soluble B vitamin, biotin is stable when heated. It is involved in the utilization of glucose, by increasing insulin action, and can be used in the control of sugar levels in diabetics. It also assists with the utilization of protein, folic acid and vitamin B12.

Biotin is synthesized in the body by the intestinal flora (bacteria) so that healthy flora are an important factor in the maintenance of correct biotin levels and the prevention of deficiency symptoms. In this respect, eggs are best eaten cooked since raw egg white is rich in avidin, a protein which binds biotin and prevents its absorption. Biotin helps to maintain the skin in a healthy condition and alleviate eczema and dermatitis. It also eases muscle aches and is reputed to prevent the hair from greying. Its deficiency symptoms include eczema and dermatitis, lack of appetite, fatigue and muscle pains. Biotin is useful in the treatment of hair and scalp conditions. For instances, it is sometimes used in case of hair loss, and a scalp condition in infants known as seborrheic dermatitis appears to improve with biotin supplements. The best natural sources of biotin are brewer's yeast, liver, brown rice, nuts, egg yolk, milk and fruits. The recommended daily dosage is between 150 and 300 mcg. The body's requirement of biotin increases during pregnancy and lactation.

BIRCH, WHITE BIRCH *(BETULA ALBA)*

Also known as the paper birch because of its bark which separates into sheets almost like paper, this is a tall slender tree which grows wild in northern Europe and North America. Its leaves and bark are astringent, diuretic, and promote perspiration and infusions of the leaves are claimed to dissolve kidney stones and eliminate gravel. Birch can also stimulate kidney functions and help with the elimination of uric acid. A decoction of the leaves provides a mild sedative when taken at bedtime. The decoction is made with one tablespoonful of fresh leaves boiled in half a cup of water.

This should be left to steep for two hours, after which half a teaspoonful of bicarbonate of soda should be added. An infusion can be made with one tablespoonful of leaves soaked in half a cup of hot water. Available from larger herbalists.

BIRTH CONTROL PILLS

Birth control pills are known to deplete several important vitamins in the body such as B6, folic acid and B12. Prolonged use of oral contraceptives, can create typical deficiency symptoms of these nutrients such as weight gain, oedema, allergies, anaemia, fatigue, depression, and even loss of sex drive. To prevent such symptoms, long-term users of the pill would do well to supplement their diets with these vitamins.

BIRTHWORT (*ARISTOLOCHIA CLEMATITIS*)

A perennial plant which grows wild in hedges and along fences, both its roots and clustered flower heads can be used for medicinal purposes. The ancient Egyptians used the plant as a remedy for snake bite, and infusions of the roots have traditionally been used to heal ulcers and also to arrest tumours in animals. In addition, infusions of the root and flowers will stimulate perspiration, act as a diuretic, reduce fever, and stimulate delayed menstruation. Available from larger health food stores and herbalists. Also incorporated in nutritional formulas.

BISHOP WEED (*Ammi Visnaga*)

A Middle Eastern herb commonly used in Yemenite and other Arab folk medicine, it contains the glycoside khellin, which has been found to reduce the pain of kidney stones by relieving muscle spasms due to stone pressure. It is also known to alleviate the pain of angina pectoris by dilating the arteries of the heart. Available from larger herbalists.

BITTER MELON (*Momordica charantia*)

A tropical fruit, also known as balsam pear, bitter melon is a vegetable widely cultivated in Asia, Africa and South America. The fresh juice or the extract of the unripe fruit have been found in various studies to have a blood sugar lowering effect. As such, bitter melon is extensively used in folk medicine as a treatment for diabetes.

Bitter melon contains several compounds that have anti-diabetic properties. One of them, charantin, is an efficient sugar-lowering agent composed of mixed steroids. Another active ingredient, momordica, is a polypeptide (protein) which reduces blood sugar levels, in much the same way as insulin, when injected into insulin-dependent diabetics. Drinking 50–60 ml of the juice has also shown positive results in clinical trials. Available from larger health food stores and herbalists.

BLACKBERRY (*Rubus Villosus*)

A perennial plant that grows wild and is also cultivated. Blackberry leaf infusions have astringent and blood-building properties. They have long been used as a folk remedy to treat diarrhoea and anaemia.

They also have tonic and decongestant properties and can relieve symptoms of enteritis. A tea made from the dried root can help relieve water retention (oedema).

Available from supermarkets and grocers.

BLACK COHOSH ROOT *(Cimicifuga Racemosa)*

A perennial plant, native to North America which grows wild from Maine to Missouri, mainly on hillsides. Infusions and decoctions of the root are astringent, diuretic and anti-spasmodic, and will assist with the release of phlegm from respiratory system, stimulate delayed menstrual flow and ease painful menstruation. They can also be used to reduce inflammations and increase sweating, and have been used to alleviate rheumatism and bronchitis. The American Indians used Black Cohosh to treat female complaints such as the hot flushes of menopause, as well as for rheumatism.

Incorporated in nutritional formulas.

BLACKCURRANT *(Ribes Nigrum)*

Best grown in northern regions where the weather is generally cool and humid, blackcurrants were traditionally used, much like blackberries, to prepare delicious drinks, teas or home-made syrups. However, in the recent years, the oil of the blackcurrant seed has been found to be beneficial in skin care, improving skin softness and suppleness. Blackcurrant seed oil contains essential fatty acids and is one of the richest sources of gamma-linolenic acid (**GLA**) – in fact it contains about 15 per cent more GLA than **evening primrose oil** – and is sold under different brand names in health food shops in capsules of various potencies.

BLACK NIGHTSHADE *(SOLANUM NIGRUM)*

An annual which grows wild on sea cliffs and cultivated land, mainly in England and Wales, although it has been introduced into Scotland and Ireland. It contains several alkaloids, including atropine, solanine and solasodine, a derivative of diosgenin from which plant steroids are made.

Caution: All nightshades (see BELLADONNA) are highly poisonous and must only be used under strict medical supervision.

BLOOD CLOTTING

Normal blood clotting is necessary for healing wounds. Vitamin K promotes blood clotting and is used to prevent or control internal bleedings and reduce excessive menstrual flow. However, excessive blood clotting is dangerous and can result in coronary thrombosis and thrombophlebitis, the main causes of heart attacks, as well as strokes. The risk of excessive blood clotting is increased by nutrient deficiencies, alcohol and excess **arachidonic acid (*AA*)**, an essential fatty acid prevalent in meat, dairy, eggs and peanuts. A vegetarian diet can therefore be beneficial in such cases. A reduction in blood–clotting can be induced by foods such as garlic, onion and fish (such as salmon, mackerel and sardines), and the use of supplements such as **vitamin E, calcium, evening primrose oil, omega–3 fatty acids** (MaxEPA), **lecithin, kelp** and **octacosanol**, contained in **wheat germ oil**.

BLOOD SUGAR

Since the body burns sugar (**glucose**) for energy, it is imperative that a consistently adequate blood sugar level is maintained in order to retain a feeling of well-being – an ideal blood sugar level is between 90 and 100 mg glucose per 100 cc of blood. At this level we are energetic and feel good, but when the level drops to 70 mg, hunger, fatigue and irritability set in. At levels below this, exhaustion, dizziness, heart palpitations and nausea are common.

The pancreas is the major sugar regulator and the body has a complicated hormonal balancing mechanism which keeps blood sugar at a fairly constant level. When the sugar level rises too high, the pancreas secretes insulin which converts glucose to glycogen. When the blood sugar drops too low, the pancreas secretes glucagon and the adrenal glands secrete adrenalin, two hormones that convert glycogen back to glucose. However, if this balancing mechanism gets out of order, it can produce either low blood sugar (hypoglycaemia) or high blood sugar (diabetes). Factors that can affect the blood sugar balance include an excessive use of white sugar, prolonged stress and nutrient deficiencies. Elimination of white sugar from the diet, together with supplements of the B-complex vitamins, chromium picolinate or GTF chromium, zinc and brewer's yeast will help to restore and stabilize the blood sugar to a more acceptable level.

BLUE FLAG (IRIS VERSICOLOR)

Also known as flag lily or wild iris, blue flag is a perennial iris which is a native of American swamps and wetlands, but nowadays can be found planted in gardens throughout

Britain. Infusions of the root are diuretic and can be used as a tonic, to assist with purifying the blood, expelling intestinal worms and the relief of vaginal infections. Due to its diuretic properties, blue flag was traditionally used to treat oedema. It is also recommended for migraines caused by stomach disorders. Available from larger herbalists.

BLUE GUM TREE SEE EUCALYPTUS

BLUE-GREEN ALGAE *(APHANIZOMENON FLOS-AQUAE)*

Blue-green algae, or AFA, is one of the fastest growing items in the health food market. This unique algae, which is found in Upper Klamath Lake in South Oregon, is considered to be a perfect 'green food' as it contains 60 per cent high quality protein, together with all the essential amino acids required for full utilization. It is the richest known source of chlorophyll, which is a blood purifier, is high in beta carotene and contains a vast array of vitamins, minerals and trace elements, including high concentration of vitamin B12. AFA has been found to have many beneficial effects and regular users report experiencing increased energy and mental alertness, as well as improvement in conditions such as depression, diabetes, hypoglycaemia, anaemia and Alzheimer's. AFA is available from health food shops in capsules, tablets and powder form.

Note: At the time of publication, some reports have indicated that the supplement may contain toxins linked to paralysis and long-term liver damage.

BONEMEAL

Usually derived from cattle bones, this is a calcium–phosphorus supplement which is sold in health food shops in both tablet and powder form. However, since the bonemeal **calcium** is not chelated, it is best taken with a protein meal.

BORAGE OIL

A native of the Mediterranean regions, borage (also called starflower) was brought to Britain by the Romans. The oil of borage is used as a dietary source for gamma–linolenic acid (**GLA**) and, in fact, has been found to provide a more concentrated source of GLA than the more generally used **evening primrose oil** – some batches can be as high in GLA as 20 per cent. A recent study has shown that borage oil can lower hypertension and, as a dietary supplement, has brought about a reduction in high blood pressure within a period of seven weeks. Available from health food stores.

BORON

This trace element was recently found to promote the absorption of **calcium** and **magnesium**. Boron also inter-acts with **potassium**, **vitamin D** and **methionine**, and has been found to raise in women the level of estradiol, the most active type of oestrogen. Boron can therefore be bene-ficial in menopause, when oestrogen levels drop and calcium absorption is impaired. Boron has also been found to be effective in alleviating symptoms of arthritis, especially juve-nile arthritis. Deficiency symptoms of boron include bone demineralization, brittle bones, arthritis, low oestrogen levels in menopause and reduced growth. Best natural sources of the element are fruits, vegetables and supplements – 3 mg a day provides a normal intake.

Available from health food stores.

BRAN

Bran is made up of the fibrous husks that cover grain seeds. It contains 12 per cent polysaccharides (cellulose, pectin and lignin) and also protein, fat, vitamins and minerals. Contrary to its common description as 'roughage' food, it is not irritating to the bowels. Wheat bran contains 2.5 per cent cellulose (the indigestible part) which compares favourably with apples (3.6 per cent) and grapes (7 per cent).

However, bran is not recommended so much for its nutritional value, but rather for the ability of its fibre to absorb water and give bulk to the faeces. It expands in the colon, stimulating bowel movement and elimination. High fibre diets speed up waste transit time through the colon, preventing constipation, appendicitis, diverticulosis (pockets in the colon), haemorrhoids and varicose veins, obesity and high blood pressure, cancer of the colon and coronary heart disease. With slow moving stools, unfriendly bacteria in the colon have time to convert bile acids to carcinogens, whereas fast moving stools facilitate bile excretion, reducing cholesterol, hypertension and heart attack. Wheat bran, oat bran and rice bran are among the most popular. Available from supermarkets and health food stores.

BRANCHED CHAIN AMINO ACIDS *(BCAA)*

This group contains three essential amino acids: leucine, isoleucine and valine. BCAA are essential for muscle growth and repair; also helping to heal muscle tears, sprains and tired muscles and are mostly used, therefore, by athletes and body builders. BCAA can also help to strengthen weak muscles in people after a period of being bedridden and are good stress relievers. They are available from health food stores as a food supplement.

BRASSICA

A family of vegetables which includes cabbage, broccoli, Brussels sprouts, cauliflower, turnip and kale. They are rich in vitamins and minerals, particularly sulphur, the 'beauty mineral' which produces collagen and boosts the immune system against germs and viruses. They also contain compounds with anti-cancer properties such as dithiolthiones and indoles which protect against breast and colon cancer. This family of vegetables also has a beneficial effect on the liver.

BREAST FEEDING SEE BABY, FOOD

BREWER'S YEAST

A unicellular micro-organism, brewer's yeast was originally a by-product of the brewing industry, which was grown on hops, grain or malt, and which had to be debittered. Now, due to is high nutritional value, brewer's yeast is mainly produced as a supplement. The best types are those graded 'primary'.

These are usually grown on molasses or sugar beets and are pleasant-tasting.

Brewer's yeast is a well-balanced food, containing excellent concentrations of B–complex vitamins, even including vitamin B12 in some cases. It is up to 45 per cent complete protein, containing 17 **amino acids**, including all the essential ones, and is a rich source of DNA and RNA, which together form 12 per cent of dried yeast. It also contains an abundance of minerals and trace elements. For example, it is high in **iron** and **copper**, making it helpful in the treatment of anaemia. In addition, it contains high amounts of **chromium** and **glucose tolerance factor (GTF)** which benefits diabetics and hypoglycaemics. It also contains **selenium** – in fact, some yeasts are actually grown on selenium, making them 'selenium-rich yeast'. This selenium, in particular, is easily absorbed. Initially, only small amounts of brewer's yeast should be taken on a daily basis; then, as the body adapts to it, the amounts can gradually be increased. It is available from health food shops in tablet, flake or powder form.

Caution: Brewer's yeast is contra-indicated in cases of candida (thrush).

BROCCOLI

A member of the Brassica family, it is a green vegetable that can be eaten either cooked or raw. It is exceptionally rich in nutrients, containing an abundance of sulphur, iron and chlorophyll, which purifies the blood; it is also rich in vitamins A, B complex and, especially, vitamin C. In fact, it contains more vitamin C than oranges – one cupful provides 70 mg vitamin C which can be readily absorbed and utilized by the body, unlike the synthetic vitamin.

Caution: Broccoli should be avoided in cases of thyroid deficiency, goitre or low iodine conditions, since it contains substances that inhibit the absorption of iodine.

BROMELAIN

A protein–splitting enzyme which is present in pineapple and, in fact, pineapple has traditionally been used in the Caribbean regions as meat tenderizer, which is why pineapple can combine well with meat dishes. As a supplemental digestive aid, Bromelain is available in health food shops in tablet or capsule form.

BRUSSELS SPROUTS

A member of the Brassica family of vegetables, Brussels sprouts are similar to **cabbage** in flavour and nutrient content and provide an excellent source of vitamins C, B1 and beta carotene. Similarly, they are also rich in potassium, calcium and sulphur, but unlike cabbage and broccoli, which can be enjoyed both in their raw form and cooked, Brussels sprouts are only palatable as a cooked vegetable.

BUCHU *(BOROSMA BETULINA)*

A small shrub that is native to South Africa, where its leaves are dried and used as a tea that is drunk as a tonic. It is also exported to Britain and the US, where it is recognized as an excellent herb tea for those who suffer from cystitis, urinary gravel and other urinary problems. Available from health food stores.

BUCKWHEAT, KASHA

Buckwheat is a unique alkali-forming grain (another is millet) which, when roasted, is known as 'kasha'. It is rich in fibre and silica and strengthens the intestines, which makes it a useful food in the treatment of chronic diarrhoea and dysentery. Buckwheat is noted for being a very rich source of rutin, the bioflavonoid which is known to strengthen capillaries, inhibit inner bleeding, treat and prevent piles and varicose veins and help reduce high blood pressure. Sprouted buckwheat is rich in chlorophyll, vitamins and enzymes. Available from supermarkets and health food stores.

Caution: Unlike millet, buckwheat does contain gluten and so should not be used in a gluten-free diet.

BURDOCK *(ARCTIUM LAPPA)*

A small biennial plant which grows wild in North America and Europe, its leaves, roots and seeds all have nutritional and medicinal uses. It is a diuretic and blood cleanser, promotes perspiration and stimulates digestion. In addition, it has chemical constituents that are anti-fungal, anti-bacterial and anti-tumour, making it an important herb for use in the prevention of cancerous growths.

Burdock also contains the polysaccharide inulin, which is known to reduce inflammations and, as an anti-bacterial, it can help with the treatment of staph infections.

The fresh plant is used in macrobiotic cooking. For infusions and decoctions, fresh root can be grated to a juice, or used dried.

Capsules available from health food stores. It is also incorporated in nutritional formulas and available as a dried herb from herbalists.

BUTCHER'S BROOM *(RUSCUS ACULEATUS)*

An evergreen shrub of the lily family, it is the rhizome of the plant which has medicinal properties as it contains active alkaloids that have many physiological effects. For instance, they are anti–inflammatory and can constrict blood vessels. The plant was traditionally used in treating vein disorders, both internally and externally, such as piles and varicose veins. In addition, infusions made from the rhizome are recognized as a good herbal drink for jaundice, oedema or gout.

Capsules are available from health food stores. It is also incorporated in nutritional formulas and available as a dried herb from herbalists.

BUTTER, BUTYRIC ACID

Butter consists mainly of saturated fat and cholesterol, containing only a scant amount of protein and essential fatty acids. As such, it can raise cholesterol levels and contribute to heart disease, although in this respect it is less harmful than standard margarine. For instance, butter contains 4 to 6 per cent essential fatty acids, which help to prevent heart attack, while margarine contains only 2 to 5 per cent. Butter is also a rich source of vitamin A and contains butyric acid, a short chain fatty acid which is needed for cell health and repair. As with other fats when heated above certain temperatures, butter oxidizes and decomposes, producing irritating substances in the digestive tract. For frying purposes, it is important to note that the fatty acids in butter decompose at 226F (or 108C). It is best to adjust frying temperatures accordingly, and never refry previously heated butter.

C

CABBAGE

One of the Brassica family, cabbage provides a rich source
of vitamin C – in fact, the vitamin C content of cabbage is
greater than that of oranges. It also contains a large number
of minerals, including iodine, sulphur, calcium, magnesium
and potassium. The outer leaves contain more vitamin E
and calcium than the inner leaves. If prepared as sauerkraut,
it makes an excellent food for strengthening the intestines
and promoting a healthy flora.

Cabbage is recommended in natural medicine practice
for improving digestion, treating constipation, preventing
the common cold and alleviating depression. It also contains
a factor called **vitamin U**, which is a remedy for ulcers and
raw cabbage juice has been reported to assist in the cure of
both peptic and duodenal ulcers. The recommended
method is to drink half a cup of freshly made cabbage juice
two or three times a day between meals, on an empty stomach. Many of the healing properties of cabbage as a blood
purifier are due to its high sulphur content. Grated cabbage
can also be made into a poultice to be applied externally in
the treatment of wounds, varicose veins and leg ulcers.

CADMIUM

Cadmium is a highly toxic element – as little as one-half to
one ppm in water can be toxic – and, once in the body,

cadmium displaces zinc and accumulates in the kidneys, liver and blood vessels, probably for life.

Cadmium occurs naturally in zinc ores, but is a typical environmental pollutant and since it is present in car exhaust fumes, it pollutes the air of all major cities. It is also found in cigarette smoke – a 20-pack of cigarettes contains 20 mg of cadmium, half of which is absorbed during smoking. Nickel–cadmium battery plants are well-known sources of pollution, as are incinerators of discarded cars, and zinc and copper smelting plants. Cadmium is also contained in phosphate fertilizers, via which it can contaminate vegetation. Another source of cadmium is drinking water from corroded pipes, especially soft water which increases corrosion.

Cadmium is one of the major contributors to high blood pressure, atherosclerosis, strokes and heart attacks. Emphysema patients have been found to have more cadmium in their kidneys and liver than healthy people – cigarette smoking, in particular, has been associated with emphysema because of the cadmium content of cigarette smoke.

Nutritional protection from the toxic effects of cadmium can be provided by zinc, which replaces cadmium, and by large doses of vitamin C.

CAFFEINE, COFFEE

Caffeine is the most prevalent stimulant in Western society since it is present in coffee, tea, cocoa, chocolate, colas, as well as many of the over-the-counter stimulants and drugs such as analgesics. It has been estimated that the average daily caffeine consumption per person is between 150–225 mg, 75 per cent of which comes from coffee. A cup of coffee contains between 50 and 150 mg of caffeine, while a cup of tea contains about 50 mg and a 12-ounce can of cola contains about 35 mg.

However, caffeine consumption in heavy coffee drinkers is far higher – in some cases this can be anything up to 7,500 mg a day! The excessive and prolonged intake of coffee can cause 'caffeinism' symptoms such as anxiety, nervousness, insomnia, depression, constipation, frequent urination, duodenal ulcers, high cholesterol, hypertension and heart disease; it is also believed to be involved in a proneness to breast lumps, while coffee drinking during pregnancy is thought to increase the risk of miscarriage. People who are sensitive to 'caffeinism' can exhibit some of these symptoms with as little as two cups of coffee a day.

In addition, caffeine inhibits absorption of iron, promoting anaemia, it can create deficiencies of inositol and calcium as it interferes with their absorption, and, since it raises the cholesterol level, it can increase the proneness to heart attack.

However, there are two external applications in which coffee can be beneficial: a poultice of wet ground coffee can help to heal bruises and alleviate the effects of insect bites, and it can also be used therapeutically in enemas.

CALCIUM

Calcium is the most abundant mineral in the human body, with almost all of it – 99 per cent – found in the bones and the teeth, or helping to build bone mass and preventing osteoporosis. However, the remaining 1 per cent, which is in blood, is of paramount importance to the body as it normalizes nerve and muscle function, regulates heartbeat, enables blood clotting, helps to maintain a proper acid–alkaline balance, induces sleep and promotes skin health.

Unfortunately, absorption of calcium in the body is very inefficient and there are a number of factors needed for its proper absorption, including stomach acid (HCl), vitamins A, C and D, magnesium and protein. In addition, while regular exercise will promote calcium deposition in bones, a sedentary lifestyle depletes it, causing porous bones. Pregnant and menopausal women, especially, are very vulnerable to calcium deficiencies and bone loss unless they take calcium supplements. Older men can also be prone to calcium deficiency and also people with digestive disorders, such as ulcers or Crohn's disease, because of the accompanying reduction in stomach secretions. Coffee, alcohol, soft drinks, diuretics, antacids and excess protein can all deplete calcium levels.

Deficiency symptoms include brittle bones, tooth decay, nervousness, muscle aches, leg cramps, excessive menstrual flow and impaired growth. A high supplement of calcium (1–2 g per day) not only helps to reverse bone loss (osteoporosis), but also treats conditions such as high cholesterol levels and hypertension. Among the best natural sources are dairy products, sesame seeds, soya beans, peanuts, green vegetables, sunflower seeds, bone–marrow soups and calcium tablets. Calcium citrate is considered to be the best absorbed form of calcium, and has the least risk of developing kidney stones.

The normal recommended daily allowance of calcium for adults is 800 mg, while the recommended daily dosage for pregnant and lactating women is 1,200 mg. However, many experts recommend higher doses of up to 1.5 g per day.

CALCIUM ASCORBATE

This is an acid–free form of vitamin C in which calcium is used to buffer the acidity of vitamin C.

CALORIE

A calorie is a unit of energy that represents the amount of heat required to raise the temperature of one gram of water by one Celsius degree. In terms of human nutrition, calories are a measurement of the energy produced when food is metabolized by the body. Thus, calorific values denote the amount of heat energy yielded by different foods, and are usually expressed on food labels as Kcal (kilo calorie) units.

Different types of foods supply different amounts of calories – for instance, proteins and carbohydrates provide 4 Kcal per gram each, while fats provide 9 Kcal per gram – and the calories received from food are 'burned' in the course of our daily activities. Thus, in a perfect situation, the amount of calories consumed from food should equal the amount of calories spent. In such a case, the energy flow is balanced. However, when more calories are eaten than spent, the excess calories are stored as fat and the result is overweight. Conversely, by eating fewer calories than the body requires will result in a loss of weight. One pound of body fat equals 3,500 calories, but the daily calorie require-ment for individuals varies greatly according to their age, sex, body type, genetic predisposition and lifestyle.

However, not all calories are created equal. Slimmers should remember that sugar calories are more fattening than protein or complex carbohydrate calories.

CALORIE RESTRICTED DIETS

Calorie restricted diets with proper supplementation have been found to extend the life span of laboratory animals. Young animals restricted to 60 per cent of their normal food intake, lived up to 50 per cent longer than animals with no food limits. In addition, the animals who were eating less were much healthier and looked youthful into their old age. The anti-ageing effects of calorie restriction were discovered as early as 1934, but until recently it was not known how this works. However, research has now shown that food restriction retards the ageing of the pineal gland. This is the gland that produces **melatonin**, a hormone that greatly influences our health and well-being, and production of which decreases with age. Studies done by life insurance companies have shown that, statistically, overweight people have the shortest life span while those whose weight is just below the average, have the longest life span.

CAMOMILE (*MATRICARIA CHAMOMILLA*)

An annual plant, which is native to the Mediterranean countries, it is now widely cultivated in more temperate regions such as the British Isles. The herb has long been used for its calming effect and has also been found beneficial in the treatment of indigestion, colic, spasms, stomach cramps and insomnia. Camomile also has antiseptic properties and can be used for the alleviation of inflammations of the digestive tract. In addition, it is used in mouthwashes and gargles, as well as in sitz baths to alleviate haemorrhoids, and in enema solutions. The dried flowers are very popular as a herb tea, which is obtainable either as tea bags or loose, in bulk. Available from supermarkets and health food stores.

CANOLA OIL

This is produced from the canola variety of rapeseed which has a high content of a monounsaturated fat, oleic acid. Canola oil is often recommended because of its low saturated fat content (6 per cent), its omega-3 fatty acids (10 per cent) and especially for its monounsaturates (60 per cent), which make it safer and healthier than most other vegetable oils. The oil is used by food processing companies to make cooking oil and products such as margarine and salad dressings.

CAPRYLIC ACID

A naturally occurring fatty acid, it is commercially derived from coconut oil. Caprylic acid has been found to have antifungal properties and is used to treat candidiasis. It is absorbed in the intestines, and the tablets should be enteric-coated, or time-release, to protect them during their passage through the stomach, until they reach the intestines. Available from health food stores.

CARAWAY *(Carum Carvi)*

A biennial cultivated herb, its seed are commonly used for flavouring foods, especially bread. Caraway can stimulate the appetite, relieve flatulence and improve digestion. It can also promote the onset of menstruation and alleviate uterine cramps. The seeds can also be used to prepare an infusion, using one teaspoonful of crushed seeds boiled in half a cup of water. Available from supermarkets or health food stores.

CARBOHYDRATES

Carbohydrates are organic chemical compounds whose molecule contains carbon, hydrogen and oxygen. They are the main food group for supplying the body's energy and as such are known as 'energy food'.

Carbohydrates come in several varieties and types: monosaccharides, or simple sugars, which include glucose, fructose and galactose, found in fruits and honey; disaccharides, the more complex sugars which include sucrose (in cane and beet sugar), lactose (in milk) and maltose (in malted barley); and finally, polysaccharides, or complex carbohydrates, which include starch, cellulose and glycogen.

All carbohydrates (except cellulose) are ultimately converted in the body to glucose. This is the sole usable form of energy, and the body depends on a continuous supply of it for all its activities, mental and physical.

Carbohydrates yield 4 calories per gram. The most widely used carbohydrate is sucrose, or refined sugar. Calories derived from sugar through sweetened foods and drinks have been termed 'empty calories', because these foods lack the essential vitamins, minerals and other nutrients that accompany whole natural fruits in nature, such as the sugar cane and beets from which they are derived. Excess consumption of refined sugar can have many detrimental effects, from tooth decay, obesity and fatigue to high cholesterol levels, hypoglycaemia and diabetes. Sugar is also a stressing food.

CARDAMOM *(ELETTARIA CARDAMOMUM)*

A perennial plant which grows wild in India, it also now cultivated in other tropical areas of the world. The seeds of the plant, which are enclosed in fruity pods, have both medicinal and culinary uses. Cardamom is known as a carminative, relieving flatulence, stimulating the stomach and aiding digestion. However, it is mainly used as a cooking spice or for flavouring drinks and medicines. In Arab countries it is commonly added to coffee. Widely available.

CARNITINE, L-CARNITINE

A non-essential amino acid which plays a part in the utilization of fats in the body, it also helps to transport fatty acids to the mitochondria, the tiny power plants in the cells that convert fat to energy. Thus, by reducing triglycerides level, supplemental carnitine can help to reduce angina pectoris attacks and provide protection from heart failure. Carnitine also inhibits the development of fatty liver disease induced by alcohol, and assist with weight loss, fighting fatigue and the release of more energy. Available from health food stores.

CAROB *(CERATONIA SILIQUA)*

Also called locust bean, carob has been known since biblical times as St John's bread. The carob is an evergreen tree, native to Mediterranean countries, which is found both wild and cultivated. The carob produces long pods containing both gum and seeds, both of which have culinary and medicinal uses.

The gum, which has a flavour similar to cocoa, is rich in natural sugars such as galactomannan, calcium and minerals. Carob powder, produced from the dried gum, is now increasingly used commercially as a chocolate substitute in confectionery and biscuits for people allergic to chocolate.

The food industry also uses carob as an emulsifier and stabiliser (E410) in many foods, such as ice creams, soups and salad dressings. Carob powder is available in health food stores as a cocoa substitute for home baking purposes.

CAROTENOIDS

This is the common name for several hundred plant pigments which are powerful **antioxidants**. Carotenoids absorb the dangerous rays of the sun that produce free radicals in plants. These free radicals are extremely harmful, not only to plants, but to humans too where they can cause the degenerative diseases of ageing such as heart disease, cancer and arthritis. Thus, the inclusion in the diet of plenty of fresh fruits and vegetables containing carotenoids can help to provide protection from the damaging effects of free radicals. Some carotenoids, such as alpha, **beta** and gamma carotenes, are also provitamin A precursors. Non-provitamin A dietary carotenoids include lycopene, lutein and zeaxanthin. There are indications that lycopene, found mainly in tomatoes, may help to lower the risks of prostate cancer development, while alpha carotene, found in carrots, may provide protection from some forms of cancer. Lutein and zeaxanthin are thought to prevent macular degeneration, a leading cause of blindness in the elderly. Carotenoids are increasingly available as nutritional supplements, particularly in formulas.

CARRAGEENAN

Carrageenan is a jellying compound extracted from red seaweeds (algae). Traditionally, the Irish extracted it from Irish

Moss (chondrus crispus) and used it as a food and remedy for respiratory diseases. Commercially, carrageenan was not produced until the Second World War, when an alternative to the Japanese **agar** (E406) was needed.

Carrageenan is composed of several hydrocolloids, rather than a single substance. It consists of varying amounts of calcium, magnesium, ammonium, potassium and sodium salts of sulphate esters of galactose and 3,6-anhydro-galactose copolymers. The carrageenan used in food has a high molecular weight and comprises all the long chain molecules of the copolymers. This is termed 'Food Grade Carrageenan'. Degraded carrageenan has low molecular weight with no jellying properties.

Carrageenan comes in the form of dried, translucent mucilage that swells in cold water, dissolving partially to make a jelly. It is used (in low concentrations of up to 1 per cent) in the food industry as a stabilizing, thickening, suspending and jellying agent. For example, it is extensively used as a stabilizer of milk proteins in such products as ice cream, milk shakes and milk chocolate (E407).

Degraded carrageenan, which is not permitted in food use, was found to cause ulcerative colitis and tumours in animals. This is why the use of degraded carrageenan was forbidden by EEC statutory regulations, which has led to public confusion about the safety of carrageenan. However, although carrageenan undergoes some degradation in the acid environment of the stomach, small amounts do not appear to cause any harm; it is only in large amounts that is suspected of being a health hazard.

CARROT

A common root vegetable, it is one of the richest sources of beta carotene, a vitamin A precursor. Carrots are also an excellent source of vitamins B1 and B2 and of the minerals potassium, sodium and silicon. Carrots have been reported to help night vision, inhibit cataracts, treat indigestion and protect against cancer. They are also thought to be useful in treating infections of the lung, digestive system and urinary tract. Regular inclusion of carrots in the diet, either raw or cooked, can improve skin appearance and calcium absorption, while cooked carrots can benefit people with weak digestion. Carrot juice, which is pleasant on its own, provides a good basis for the addition of other less palatable juices such as celery or beet.

Caution: It is recommended that the intake of carrot juice should be limited to no more than four cups a day since over-consumption can cause yellowing of the skin, a condition known as xanthosis.

CARTILAGE, SHARK AND BOVINE

Sharks have long been known for their high resistance to disease and wound healing ability. Unlike other vertebrates, the shark's skeleton in composed of a special cartilage, and it is to this that its healing properties are attributed.

The cartilage of the shark has been found to have strong anti-cancer and anti-inflammatory effects which, when used on humans, can help to restore flexibility to arthritic joints and inhibit the growth of malignant tumours. Recently, attention has also been focused on bovine cartilage which appears to have similar properties. Most of the studies done have confirmed its efficacy and, in fact, suggest that much lower doses of bovine cartilage are required to be effective, making its use more practical than that of shark's cartilage. Available from health food stores.

CASCARA SAGRADA *(RHAMNUS PURSHIANA OR RHAMNUS CATHARTICUS IN THE UK)*

A small tree or shrub which is native to North America, its Spanish name *cascara sagrada* means 'sacred bark', and it is the bark of the tree that has traditionally been used as a herbal laxative. In some countries it is dispensed as a prescription herb and its active ingredients include certain glycosides (anthraquinones) and bitter principles, which act on the bowels, increasing their movement, and promoting evacuation. Cascara is generally considered safe. However, when used in excessive dosages or over prolonged periods of time, it can cause toxic reactions. Cascara is available in several forms, such as the dried herb and as an extract, and it is now becoming increasingly used in laxative formulas sold in health food shops.

CASHEW NUT

A bean-shaped nut that grows on a tropical evergreen tree, it was originally native to Central America, but is now also grown in India, Brazil and several African countries. It is rich in protein, minerals, especially magnesium, some B vitamins and fat, and has become increasingly popular in recent years as a snack food. It is also marketed as 'cashew butter'. Due to its high fat content, it is better eaten raw than roasted.

Caution: The cashew tree is related to poison ivy, and

the shell of the cashew nut contains an irritating poison which, if touched, can sometimes cause skin blistering. However, this poison is only present in the shells – the kernels, which are normally sold shelled, are harmless in this respect.

CAT'S CLAW *(UNCARIA TOMENTOSA)*

A herb which originates from the Amazon rainforest, it has been hailed in recent years as an immune system booster and has been found to be particularly beneficial in the treatment of cancer and AIDS. The herb is currently being researched in several countries, with studies checking its possible benefits in the treatment of arthritis, allergies, ulcers, cancer and acne, and there has been an increasing demand for cat's claw in health food shops where it is sold as a tea and as capsules.

CATNIP *(NEPETA CATARIA)*

Also known as catmint, this is an aromatic perennial herb of the mint family. Its leaves can be used to make an effective infusion for upset stomach, colic and flatulence. It can also be used in enemas. Available from health food stores, incorporated in nutritional formulas and available from herbalists.

CAULIFLOWER

A very nutritious vegetable of the Brassica family, it is rich in vitamins C, B1 and B2 and a good source of calcium, magnesium, phosphorus, potassium and sulphur. It is usually cooked but can be eaten raw, or is occasionally pickled. It should be stored in the refrigerator, and when selecting cauliflower, look for fresh compact heads, with no discoloration; if the buds are spread out or spotted, this means that the cauliflower is old or has been exposed too long to the sun. People with sensitive digestion may find that the raw vegetable causes flatulence or bloating and, in such cases, it is advisable to slightly cook or sauté the cauliflower.

CAYENNE PEPPER *(CAPSICUM FRUTESCENS)*

Originally, a perennial plant native to the tropical regions of Central America, it is now cultivated elsewhere as an annual. The fruits, or hot peppers, commonly known as chillis, contain capsaicin, a stimulant which helps to control pain and dissolve blood clots. Chillis can stimulate the appetite and digestion, release phlegm and increase sweating and resistance to colds. In moderation, powdered chillis can help heal stomach and duodenal ulcers, promoting tissue growth through the release of histamine. Cayenne pepper is also effective in the treatment of ailments as diverse as arthritis, asthma, diabetes, high blood pressure, kidney infections, sinusitis and other respiratory problems, as well as reputedly providing a remedy for hangovers.

CELERY

A popular vegetable which is related to carrots and parsley, it probably originated in the Mediterranean regions. The vegetable is available all year round and provides a good source of vitamins A, B1 and B2, as well as the minerals calcium, phosphorus and silicon. The stalks of the plant, which are rich in iron, magnesium and carotene, are usually eaten raw in salads or with dips, or used in soups and as a garnish for other foods. They are high in roughage and when eaten between meals, can help with appetite control. On the other hand, the leaves are thought to stimulate the appetite, and also increase urination and bring on menstruation. Celery juice has been used to alleviate oedema, treat rheumatism and clear skin problems and, combined with a little lemon juice, it can help to prevent a cold developing. Both the stalks and roots are used to treat hypertension, and the seeds are used as a sedative and to relieve flatulence. A decoction of the seeds can be used as a remedy for rheumatism, bronchitis and calming frayed nerves. Dried ground celery is sold as a salt substitute for low sodium diets.

CENTAURY *(CENTAURIUM ERYTHRAEA)*

As a small annual, the herb grows wild on chalk downs and sandy soils throughout Europe. The small pink or white flowers are used as an infusion taken before meals to stimulate appetite and aid digestion by encouraging the liver to secrete bile. It can also act as a blood purifier and help to reduce fever. Applied externally, centaury is reputed to repel fleas and lice. Available from larger health food stores and herbalists.

CELLULOSE

Cellulose is a component of plant cell walls, which is indigestible and insoluble in water.

However, it has the ability to bind water and increase stool mass and weight, promoting bowel movement and elimination. Moreover, it also speeds up stool transit time, i.e. the time needed for food to travel from mouth to anus. Thus, it helps to prevent severe colon conditions such as constipation, diverticulitis and colon cancer. Small parts of cellulose ferment and degrade in the colon, and this degradation produces **short chain fatty acids** which are important for the energy metabolism of the colon. A major source of cellulose is **wheat bran.**

CHELATION

The word chelate comes from Greek 'chele', meaning 'claw', and chelation is the process by which minerals such as iron, chromium, zinc and magnesium, which are poorly absorbed, can be transported from the intestines to the bloodstream. The ions of these minerals contain electrical charges that are repelled by the cells of the membranes and, to overcome this, they have to be held ('clawed'), or bonded, by other chemicals, usually amino acids, which neutralize the ions. As a result, the minerals, now no longer electrically charged, can easily cross the intestinal wall to the bloodstream and be made available to the body.

Nowadays, most minerals marketed are 'amino acid chelates'. For example, chromium is chelated with picolinic acid and is usually sold as 'chromium picolinate'.

CHERRY

This attractive tree, which is a native of Europe and western Asia, produces beautiful clusters of small pink or white blossoms in springtime, while its fruit is well-known in natural medicine as an effective treatment for arthritis, gout and rheumatism. Cherries are rich sources of flavonoids such as anthocyanidins and proanthocyanidins which give the fruits their deep red–blue colour. These flavonoids are potent **antioxidants** that make them useful in treating a variety of inflammations by inhibiting histamine release. They protect collagen from free radical damage, help to prevent wrinkles and also reduce uric acid levels, thus benefiting gout. Half a pound of the fresh fruit a day constitutes a treatment for lowering uric acid levels and preventing attacks of gout.

CHROMIUM

Chromium is an essential micronutrient which is mostly removed from basic foods such as sugar and flour by refining. It is principally involved in the metabolism of glucose and the synthesis of fatty acids and cholesterol. It is also the central constituent of GTF, the glucose tolerance factor, which enhances the function of insulin. Chromium-rich diets and chromium supplements are therefore a must for diabetics, hypo-glycaemics and for anyone with a high cholesterol level or suf-fering from hypertension. Chromium has also been shown to assist in weight loss and to increase energy levels, fighting fatigue.

Chromium is best utilized in the form of chromium picolinate, which is an elemental chromium that is chelated (combined) with picolinic acid for better absorption. The best natural sources of chromium are brewer's yeast, raw wheat germ, meat, shellfish and clams, but supplements of chromium picolinate are recommended as a safeguard against chromium deficiency. The estimated daily requirement of the mineral for adults is 50–200 g, and for children is 20–80 g.

Available from health food stores.

CHICKWEED *(STELLARIA MEDIA)*

A common annual weed that can be found growing in almost all soils, the whole herb is useful for both culinary and medicinal purposes. Infusions of the plant relieve flatulence and constipation, and can also be used with soothing effects to bathe bruises and skin irritations. The herb can be eaten cooked as a vegetable, like spinach, or used raw in salads. The potassium in chickweed reduces food cravings, so that regular infusions taken three times a day can be beneficial to slimmers. Available from health food stores, incorporated in nutritional formulas, and from herbalists.

CHICORY *(CICHORIUM INTYBUS)*

A perennial plant which is cultivated in North America and Europe, mainly for its edible leaves and roots, it was popular with both the Ancient Egyptians and Greeks for its culinary and medicinal properties. Infusions or decoctions of the root or flowers can stimulate the appetite, aid digestion, promote bile secretion and help to relieve the pain and discomfort caused by gallstones. Dried ground chicory is used as a coffee substitute, either on its own or, combined with cereals, in cereal coffees. Available from supermarkets, grocers and health food stores.

CHILLI SEE CAYENNE PEPPER

CHLORELLA

A green fresh water algae, chlorella is now being marketed in health food shops as a food supplement. About 60 per cent of chlorella is in the form of high quality protein, about 20 per cent consists of carbohydrates and 10 per cent is fat. It contains more than twenty different vitamins and minerals, is a rich source of beta carotene and contains more vitamin B12 than beef liver. Chlorella also contains appreciable amounts of iron, iodine, zinc and cobalt. It is also one of the richest sources of chlorophyll and DNA.

Due to its richness in essential nutrients, many beneficial effects have been attributed to chlorella. It is reputed to stimulate the immune system and help to reduce the risk of some cancers; it has also been used to treat anaemia, fatigue, hypertension, diabetes and constipation. In addition, its high chlorophyll content makes chlorella a useful blood purifier.

CHLOROPHYLL

Chlorophyll is the green pigment in plants that enables photosynthesis, i.e. it enables sunshine to combine carbon dioxide with water, creating carbohydrates and oxygen. By utilizing light, chlorophyll is a primary source of plant energy. Its chemical structure is similar to haemoglobin (the red blood pigment that carries oxygen), which is why it is used in the treatment of certain anaemias.

It can promote growth, metabolism and respiration and has the ability to stimulate tissue growth and wound healing. Chlorophyll cream has been used to treat skin ulcers and when injected chlorophyll can help to reduce cholesterol levels. It is also known as a blood purifier, detoxifier and deodorizer.

Chlorophyll has many commercial and therapeutic applications. For instance, it is widely used in colouring food and cosmetics (E140) and a common brand of breath refreshing chewing gum contains chlorophyll.

CHOLESTEROL

Cholesterol is a form of alcohol (sterol) and a natural part of our body's cells, especially those of the brain and spinal cord, liver and kidneys. It is also abundant in egg yolks, butter and other fats and, because of this, it has been much maligned in the recent decades for its part in clogging arteries and causing heart attacks with dire warnings from the medical profession to avoid these foods.

However, cholesterol is vital to the well-being of the body. For example, it is needed to produce sex and steroid hormones and bile, synthesize vitamin D, form cell membranes and insulate nerves. It is so crucial, that all nucleated cells can synthesize it. The liver itself can produce up to one gram a day, when only about less than half of this is provided by an average diet.

Cholesterol comes in two main forms: LDL ('bad' cholesterol), which promotes cholesterol deposits and heart attacks, and HDL ('good' cholestrol), which protects the body from these harmful effects. Factors that raise cholesterol levels include smoking, stress, the pill, coffee, sugar, sweets and nutritional deficiencies. Levels can be lowered by supplements of niacin, vitamin B6, vitamin C, vitamin E, chromium, magnesium, manganese, lecithin, pectin and DHEA. Beneficial foods for the maintenance of optimum cholesterol levels include garlic, onions, aubergine, soybeans and green tea. Exercise is also very important.

CHOLINE

Choline is a lipotropic B vitamin. That is, it emulsifies fats and helps to transport fat globules to cells. It is needed for nerve transmission, liver function and lecithin formation. The brain uses choline to produce acetylcholine, a major neurotransmitter, which conveys brain cell messages and is vital for learning and memory. Choline reduces cholesterol and maintains healthy liver, kidneys and nerves. It also reduces oestrogen, thus decreasing the risk of breast lumps and menstrual cramps. Although choline can be produced in the body, it is now considered an essential food nutrient and choline supplements are known to enhance its beneficial effects. For example, they are used in the treatment of Alzheimer's disease and to improve memory and learning ability in students.

Deficiency symptoms of choline include fatty degeneration of the liver, nephritis (kidney disease), gallstones, high cholesterol and hypertension. Its best natural sources are egg yolk, liver, lecithin, brewer's yeast and green leafy vegetables. A recommended average daily intake is about 1000 mg. As a supplement, choline is commonly available as choline bitartrate, citrate or chloride, either on its own, or included in nutritional formulas.

CHONDROITIN SULPHATES (CS)

Chondroitin sulphates are a group of thick gelatinous materials called mucopolysaccharides or glycosaminoglycans (GAGs). These are types of water-bonded, long-chain sugars, which are formed in the body. They are found throughout the cartilage, collagen and connective tissues and help attract water into them, preserving their flexibility and protecting their matrix.

The production of chondroitin sulphates in the body decreases with age, and studies have shown that this reduction results in degeneration of joints (osteoarthritis) and thickening of artery walls. CS supplements are now available to counter osteoarthritis by helping to replenish cartilage.

CIDER VINEGAR

Cider vinegar is produced by the fermentation of fresh apple juice. It is both a food and a medicine, and used equally by naturopaths and cooks. It contains a combination of minerals, organic matter and acetic acid which provide its characteristic taste and smell.

There are many beneficial effects attributed to cider vinegar. First of all, it is a natural astringent and inhibits diarrhoea. It improves digestion in people with low stomach acid and acts as an intestinal antiseptic, inhibiting the decaying processes in the intestines. It also helps to overcome bad breath, increases blood clotting and wound healing, alleviates allergies, increases energy and promotes hair growth.

Cider vinegar does not work in the same way for everyone, but for sufferers of any of the above symptoms it is worth a trial. When used as a medicine, the normal method is to add two teaspoonfuls of the cider vinegar to a glass of water, one to three times a day, before meals. A teaspoonful of honey added to the drink will make it more palatable. Its culinary uses are many and it makes a good replacement for malt vinegar in many dishes, especially in salad dressings. Widely available.

CILANTRO SEE CORIANDER

CINNAMON (CINNAMOMUM ZEYLANICUM)

A popular spice used in cooking and for flavouring sweets and preserves, it comes from the inner bark of the cinnamon tree. Sri Lanka is the principal source of the spice, but the tree is also grown in Brazil, India, Jamaica, Java, Madagascar and Martinique. The powdered bark is used as a spice and also to make aromatic infusions.

Cinnamon is a disinfectant, stimulant and anti-flatulent. Warm cinnamon tea can be helpful for nausea, if sipped slowly. It can also be drunk as a relaxant and, especially at bedtime, to induce sleep. In Yemenite folk medicine, strong infusions of cinnamon are used to relieve menstrual cramps. Widely available as powder, the bark less so.

COCONUT

The coconut tree is thought to be native to south-east Asia and the Melanesian Islands of the Pacific Ocean but it is now grown in most of the tropical and subtropical regions of the world. Coconut contains small amounts of the B vitamins and larger amounts of minerals such as potassium, phosphorus, iron, magnesium and zinc. However, most of the fruit consists of saturated fat (92 per cent of its total fat), which makes it a good source of saturated fats for vegetarians, but a bad source of fat for people on meat-centred diets, or those with high cholesterol and triglyceride levels. Coconut is considered a tonic and is used for weakness conditions.

COD LIVER OIL

Cod liver oil, which is obtained from the livers of codfish, is rich in vitamins A and D, and in omega-3 fatty acids. As a supplement, in either capsule or liquid form, it supplies the important fatty acids EPA (eicosapentaenoic acid) and DHA (docosahexaenoic acid). EPA is used by the body to produce prostaglandins, hormone-like substances which help reduce stickiness of the blood, making it less prone to develop blood clots and thrombosis. EPA also reduces triglyceride levels and high blood pressure. These combined effects can significantly reduce the risk of heart disease, and the mortality of those who have already suffered a heart attack. DHA, a fatty acid found only in fish oil, is a vital component of the brain, and is needed for brain development, especially during the late stages of pregnancy. DHA is very important for children and nursing mothers since it affects learning ability. It also provides an important supplement to a vegetarian diet. DHA is also produced in the body from linolenic acid, which is found in linseed oil and evening primrose oil. (See also FATS)

Pure cod liver oil has been a traditional remedy for arthritis, both rheumatoid and osteoarthritis. The first written reference for its use as the best cure for arthritis was made by a Dutch doctor in 1849. Since the turn of the century modern science has been actively studying its benefits.

Cod liver oil was found to lubricate the joints and reduce the dryness and friction in the joint bones which causes the pain and inflammation of arthritis. Unlike normal fats which are first absorbed by the liver, the tiny droplets of cod liver oil go directly into the blood and can readily reach the joint linings. In these linings, cod liver oil is converted to mucin and hyaluronic acid, two by-products that thicken the joint fluid and help prevent bone friction at the joints. Cod liver oil has also gained a reputation for helping to cure various other conditions, such as dry eyes, dry ears, dry skin, bursitis, hair fall and arteriosclerosis. Recommended reading: *The New Arthritis and Common Sense* by Dale Alexander, and *Arthritis: Diets against it* by James Scala.

Cod liver oil is available from health food stores and pharmacies.

COENZYME Q10 *(CoQ10)*

CoQ10 is an essential nutrient that is found in every plant and animal cell. It is mainly supplied by food and, as its name implies, it is a vital catalyst – a spark plug in the conversion of food to energy within cells. In fact, CoQ10 releases 95 per cent of the energy required for life and, in this respect, a deficiency of this nutrient can cause fatigue, hypertension and heart disease. CoQ10 also has many other important roles: it is a strong antioxidant, protects oxidation of fats and prevents brown age spots; it strengthens and protects heart function by reducing heartbeat irregularities, hypertension and angina pectoris.

CoQ10 supplementation has been found to be very beneficial in halting gum recession, which is one of the main causes of lost teeth. It can also help to stimulate weight loss, while increasing energy and avoiding fatigue. The richest food sources of this nutrient are found in beef heart and other organ meats such as liver and kidney. Smaller amounts are contained in plants such as spinach, alfalfa, soybeans and potatoes. Supplemental capsules of CoQ10 are now widely available in health food shops.

COFFEE SEE CAFFEINE, COFFEE

COMFREY *(SYMPHYTUM OFFICINALIS)*

A perennial plant, which grows widely in Europe and North America, comfrey leaves were often added to salads. Its root, the part used medicinally, is rich in calcium and mucilaginous substances. The root is soothing and was used to provide intestinal lubrication while inhibiting germs such as E. coli. It is also rich in allantoin, a substance which promotes wound healing when applied topically in poultices. It can also be added to bath water to improve the skin complexion.

Until the 1980s, comfrey tablets and teas were available in health food shops. Due to its astringent qualities, the herb was used to halt diarrhoea and internal bleeding, and particularly to help heal gastric and duodenal ulcers. However, comfrey was then found to contain pyrroliziidine alkaloids, compounds reported to cause liver disease and cancer if taken over a long period of time. As a result, the free sale of comfrey tablets and teas was banned by the US FDA, and comfrey is now mainly available only in ointments, extracts and salves for external use.

COPPER

Copper is an abundant trace element which aids the absorption of iron. It is also involved in many enzyme activities and reduces histamine levels, alleviating allergies. Although an essential element, only very small amounts of copper are required by the body and even small excesses can be dangerous, causing disorders such as depression, arthritis, hypertension and heart attack. Among those most vulnerable in this respect are users of drinking water supplied from copper pipes, smokers, and women on the contraceptive pill. Zinc supplements can help to reduce excess copper levels, while the best natural sources are soybeans, legumes, whole wheat, prunes, liver, seafood and molasses. The normal daily requirement for adults is 2 mg.

CORIANDER (CORIANDRUM SATIVUM)

A small annual plant, which is a native of Mediterranean countries, its leaves are used for their distinctive flavour in salads and cooking. However, medicinally, the seeds are the most important part of the plant and an infusion of coriander seeds can strengthen digestion and relieve flatulence if taken after meals; it is also beneficial for arthritis and rheumatism. Up to three infusions a day can be consumed.
Widely available from supermarkets and health food stores.

CORN

Also called maize, corn is a cereal grass related to grains such as wheat, rice, oats and barley, and was used for thousands of years as a staple grain by the Indians of Central America. Its food value and wide variety of uses make it not only one of the foremost crops currently grown in the US, but also one of the most important crops in the world. Cornmeal, which has extensive culinary uses, is widely available and a vitally important ingredient in the coeliac diet.

Fresh corn on the cob has a delicate sweet flavour which

is soon lost after harvesting. It provides a good source of vitamins A, B1, B2, niacin, and minerals such as iron, copper, phosphorus and magnesium. Cornsilk, the fine tassel on the top of the corn cob, can be made into an infusion which soothes the urinary passages and acts as a diuretic. This can be very beneficial in cases of kidney stones and cystitis, but to be effective several cups of the infusion should be drunk each day.

CRANBERRY JUICE

Fresh cranberries and cranberry juice have been widely acclaimed in recent years as a treatment for bladder infections such as cystitis. A group study of people suffering with urinary tract infections found that a dose of 16 oz of cranberry juice had a beneficial effect in 73 per cent of the cases. Urinary tract infections can occur when bacteria adhere to the lining, or mucosa, of the bladder and urethra and infect it. Cranberry juice contains components that reduce the ability of bacteria to stick to the mucosa, thus preventing these infections.

Cranberry is available from health food shops in tablet or juice form. However, in many brands, the juice form contains only one-third cranberry juice mixed with water and sugar. This sweetened cranberry juice is not recommended, since sugar adversely affects the immune system.

CREATINE

A new dietary supplement in health food stores, recently creatine caused great excitement when studies showed its ability to improve athletic performance. Creatine supplementation was first used by the British field and track competitors, who won gold medals, in the 1992 Olympics in Barcelona. Shortly afterwards, US champion athletes began to use creatine supplements, and from there its use spread to the rest of the athletic world.

Creatine is not a steroid or a drug. It is a natural chemical which is synthesized in the body from the three amino acids, **arginine**, **methionine** and **glycine**. It is mainly stored in the skeletal muscles as phosphocreatine, the precursor of ATP, the body's prime energy chemical. Creatine is a part of a system that supplies immediate energy, and creatine supplements can produce a burst of energy. Creatine boosts muscle mass and builds voluminous, massive muscles, which is a great boon to body builders; it also increases energy, endurance and power, and can speed recovery, enabling frequent increase in exercise.

The richest dietary sources of creatine are meat and fish, especially beef, which contains two grams per pound. Typically, about two grams a day are normally synthesized by the body and two additional grams can come from food metabolism. To increase sport performance, creatine supplements are usually taken in five gram doses, one to four times a day, depending on whether the athlete is starting to load the muscles with creatine or is just maintaining its level. Creatine absorption is greatly improved when taken with insulin-releasing carbohydrates, such as grape juice. Vegetarians usually have a low intake of creatine.

CUCUMBER

A common garden vegetable, cucumber was originally native to southern Asia, but is now cultivated as an annual in many parts of the world. The fruit of the plant can be preserved by pickling with vinegar, but it is normally eaten raw as a popular addition to salads. Cucumber has diuretic properties, which can help to eliminate water from the body, and it also contains an enzyme that splits protein and cleanses the intestines. Cucumber juice is beneficial to internal inflammations, such as stomach and kidney inflammations or sore throat.

Cucumbers are best eaten with the skin, which is rich in chlorophyll and silicon. Externally, a blend of juiced cucumber with equal parts of glycerine and rose water makes a soothing lotion for chapped hands and lips.

CUMIN *(Cuminum Cyminum)*

Originating in the East, cumin is one of the oldest known culinary spices and is used in Asian cuisine to season curry. The plant has been grown in Mediterranean countries for many centuries; it was popular with the Romans and one of the most commonly used spices in Europe in the Middle Ages. The seeds, and their essential oils, are also used medicinally as an aid to stimulate gastric juices, increase appetite and relieve flatulence. Cumin is also said to increase milk secretion in nursing mothers. The seeds are widely available.

CURCUMIN *(Curcuma Longa)* SEE TURMERIC

D

DAMIANA *(Turnera Diffusa)*

A herb which grows wild in Mexico and is cultivated for its leaves, damiana is famous for its aphrodisiac properties. It is also a diuretic and a tonic, and is indicated for people who suffer from exhaustion, and for convalescence after a disease. Damiana is available in capsules as a supplement in health food stores.

DANDELION *(Taraxacum Officinale)*

A wild perennial plant, known for its bright yellow flower, it grows profusely throughout the temperate regions of the world. The whole plant is highly nutritious and can be used as a tonic, diuretic and mild laxative. When prepared as an infusion, it can be used to stimulate bile formation and is also said to relieve the symptoms of jaundice and gallstones. It is also useful for the relief of oedema and to cleanse the body from poisons. The fresh young leaves, which are best used before the flower forms, can be added to salads or used for juice. Available in tea bags in health food shops.

DEFICIENCY DISEASES

Nutrient deficiencies cause deficiency diseases – the reasons can be many and varied. For example, a deficiency may result from poor vitamin intake due to an unbalanced diet, poor absorption of nutrients due to low digestive juices or enzymes, crash diets, stress, smoking, alcohol, the contraceptive pill, or medication. Similarly, deficiency diseases can have many symptoms, such as: a deficiency of niacin can cause high cholesterol level; vitamin B12 deficiency can be reflected in fatigue and depression; calcium deficiency can cause painful leg cramps; vitamin C deficiency can cause bleeding and inflamed gums; vitamin B6 deficiency can cause kidney stones, allergies and morning sickness in pregnancy.

To avoid or correct nutrient deficiencies, it is best to balance the diet with fresh unprocessed food, and the addition of food supplements such as vitamins, minerals, trace elements, enzymes and amino acids. Determining specific supplementation should always be done in consultation with a qualified nutritionist. However, for general maintenance purposes multivitamin formulas can be taken according to doses prescribed on labels.

Caution: Some nutrients, especially in higher potencies, can cause reactions in sensitive persons. The use of higher potencies requires professional advice.

DESICCATED LIVER

This is dried beef liver which is available as tablets, capsules or powder for use as a food supplement. Desiccated liver is a rich source of the B- complex vitamins, as well as vitamins A and D. It also contains minerals such as iron, calcium, copper and phosphorus, together with protein and cholesterol. Desiccated liver is good for anaemia, weakness and particularly in the alleviation of stress. The best products are those made from organically-grown Argentinian beef liver.

DEVIL'S CLAW *(Harpagophytum Procumbens)*

A native of Namibia, this thorny plant has been found to reduce cholesterol and uric acid levels and is indicated in folk medicine for a variety of conditions, especially for gout and arthritis. It is available in health food stores in tablet form.

DHEA *(dehydroepiandrosterone)*

An abundant hormone that is synthesized by the body from cholesterol. However, cholesterol levels tend to increase with age, while DHEA levels tend to drop, and this decline signals the onset of age-related diseases. DHEA deficiencies have been implicated in diseases such as diabetes, hypertension, coronary heart disease, various cancers, and even obesity.

DHEA is now available in health food shops as a supplement, and it has been found to be beneficial in many conditions including stress relief, the treatment of diabetes, the lowering of fat and cholesterol levels. In addition, it appears to be of benefit to overweight people and those prone to heart disease, aiding in the reduction of mortality rates from heart attacks. DHEA is still being researched for further benefits.

DIETARY FIBRE see FIBRE

DILL *(Anethum Graveolens)*

An aromatic garden herb which is widely grown for its

culinary and medicinal properties. Both the leaves and seeds of the plant can be used – the young leaves to add flavour and nutrients to salads or soups and the seeds prepared as an infusion. Dill tea can relieve flatulence, strengthen digestion and stimulate appetite; it can help an upset stomach.

Available from supermarkets and grocers.

DLPA SEE PHENYLALANINE

DNA SEE NUCLEIC ACIDS

DOLOMITE

A mineral rock that is composed of calcium and magnesium carbonates, it is sold in health food stores as dolomite tablets which contain approximately two-thirds calcium and one-third magnesium. Dolomite tablets are strong alkalines and can supplement both calcium and magnesium. The tablets can help to overcome stomach acidity when taken after a meal or during a heartburn. For a quicker effect, dolomite powder is preferable, or two or three tablets crushed in the mouth before swallowing.

In the early 1980s, the US FDA cautioned the public to limit its use of dolomite because of a suspected high content of lead in dolomite tablets. Recent studies involving 70 brands of calcium supplements indicated that dolomite does not contain more lead than several other types of calcium. However, dolomite should be used by adults only, since children under 6 years of age are less able to tolerate lead than adults. It is best to buy dolomite packaged under a reputable brand name which declares its purity.

DONG QUAI

A Chinese herb, the leaves of which have been used in
China for centuries in the treatment of women's complaints, it has now been rediscovered by the West and found
to have a balancing effect on oestrogen activity and a tonic
effect on the uterus. Dong quai is used to treat female conditions such as the hot flushes of menopause, pre-menstrual
tension and vaginal dryness. It is also used to promote a
healthy pregnancy and delivery. It is available in health food
shops in capsule form, either on its own or combined with
other herbs.

DOPAMINE

This is one of the most important neurotransmitters, which
are the brain chemicals that convey messages between nerve
cells. Using dopamine as a neurotransmitter (dopaminergic
system), the nerve cells release hormone needed not only
for growth and healing, but also for the proper functioning
of the immune system in later life. Dopamine deficiency has
been found in some PMS sufferers as it suppresses the fluid
retention hormone and stimulates elimination of water and
salt. Inadequate levels of dopamine have been shown to
result in Parkinson's disease with symptoms such as uncon-
trollable tremors of the limbs. An effective treatment in
many cases is L–dopa, an amino acid which is converted in
the brain to dopamine (and norepinephrine).

E

ECHINACEA *(Echinacea Angustifolia)*

A perennial herb, native to North America, echinacea was traditionally used by the American Indians for a variety of conditions, from colds to snake bites. It was considered to be a blood purifier, analgesic and antiseptic. Another variety, Echinacea purpurea, was used in Europe for similar purposes.

The root, flowers and leaves of the plant contain many ingredients that boost the activity of the immune system and it is this property that enables echinacea to be helpful in such a variety of conditions. For instance, it can help build up resistance to colds and infections and has been found to increase the number and activity of the white blood cells of the immune system, which fight cancer cells. Due to its wide-ranging effects on the immune system, echinacea is also recommended in cases of herpes, throat infections, vaginal yeast infections, urinary tract infections, inflammatory diseases and bronchitis. The herb has recently become increasingly popular and is now available as a supplement in health food stores.

Caution: Echinacea is contra-indicated for auto-immune diseases such as AIDS or multiple sclerosis.

EGGPLANT SEE AUBERGINE

EGGS

Eggs furnish more nutrients per calorie than any other animal food except milk. Eggs contain about 73 per cent water, 6 grams protein, 5.75 grams fat and 0.45 grams carbohydrates.

Eggs are considered the most nearly perfect source of utilised protein. Eggs are low in fat, rich in vitamin A, low in calories and economical. They contain an outstandingly balanced nutrition with many B vitamins (B1, B2, B6, B12, niacin and pantothenic acid), and with many minerals and trace elements like iron, zinc, selenium, phosphorus, calcium, magnesium, potassium and especially sulfur. Egg yolk is a rich source of the important sulphur – containing amino acids, cysteine and methionine, which help build up immunity against disease.

For many years eggs were maligned as contributing to an elevated cholesterol level. It is true that egg yolks contain 275 mg of cholesterol but this is balanced by an abundance of lecithin (1, 700 mg), which emulsifies cholesterol and a vast number of other nutrients which help metabolise it. The only people who should avoid eggs are those with the condition known as hyperlipoproteinemia who should avoid all cholesterol-containing foods.

Note: raw egg white contains avidin, a protein which binds the B vitamin **biotin** and prevents its absorption.

ELDER, BLACK ELDER *(Sambucus Nigra)*

This small perennial tree, which is native to Europe, is instantly recognizable in early summer for its masses of pungent white flowers which later develop into small black berries. The leaves, blossoms, root and berries of the elder have all had their uses in European folk medicine for centuries.

Elder contains an abundance of active ingredients such as flavonoids, alkaloids and glycosides, which have many beneficial effects, particularly as anti-inflammatories, diuretics, blood vessel dilators, blood purifiers and mild laxatives.

Throughout history, a tea made of elder flowers has been used to alleviate lung infections, rheumatism, measles and scarlet fever and many herbalists still favour a strong elder blossom tea to treat colds, flu or fever, with added peppermint leaves and ginger root. Elder also encourages sweating – a boon in the treatment of colds. Nowadays, elder is also popular as a blood purifier, in cleansing fasts for building immunity and in weight reduction regimes. It is available in health food stores as a syrup, or as tablets or capsules.

ELECTROLYTES

This is a common name for dietary minerals which, in solution, can conduct electricity. These electrically charged particles, which are present throughout the body, are involved in many activities, such as regulating water retention within and out of the cells. Examples include the bulk minerals **potassium**, **sodium** and chloride.

ELM, SLIPPERY ELM *(ULMUS FULVA)*

A large deciduous tree which is native to North America, decoctions of the bark and leaves have long been a folk remedy there for many disorders. Since elm is astringent and abundant in mucilaginous matter, which lubricates and soothes mucus membranes, the decoctions are used mainly to soothe inflammations of the throat, stomach, intestines, urinary tract and lungs. Elm is also highly recommended in the treatment of stomach or duodenal ulcers. 'Slippery Elm Food' is very nutritious and, mixed with milk, it is easily digestible for people with sensitive stomachs. Externally, elm powder can be applied to cold sores, boils and burns. Elm powder and Slippery Elm Food are available in health food shops.

ENZYMES

Found in all animals and plants, enzymes are complex proteins which act as catalysts. That is, they act as agents to speed up biochemical reactions in the body, which would otherwise not take place, or that take place so slowly they appear not to be occurring. Various types of enzymes sustain life in a number of ways. For example, without digestive enzymes, digestion of food is inconceivable, and without antioxidant enzymes we could not survive for very long.

Apart from their amino acid structure, various enzymes also contain minerals and vitamins with which they co-operate as 'co-enzymes'. Enzymes can, for example, enable sugar and fat to burn at normal body temperatures, or combine oxygen and hydrogen to produce water in a reaction which would otherwise be explosive.

Each enzyme can perform only one specific chemical reaction and thousands of enzymes work in harmony to enable all the physiological activities in our bodies, from digestion to wound healing, to take place. The liver itself produces over a thousand different enzymes, but the lack of even one enzyme can break the chain of biochemical reactions, causing imbalances which are reflected as allergies, nutrient deficiencies and deficiency diseases.

The secretion of enzymes in the body declines with age, and enzyme supplementation is highly recommended, particularly after the age of 40. Various digestive enzyme supplements from both animal and vegetable origins are available in health food stores. Some, like betaine HCl, help people with low stomach acid, others such as papain and bromelain are protein-splitting enzymes, and pancreatin tablets contain various enzymes that split protein, starch and fat for a comprehensive enzymatic action.

ERGOT *(CLAVICEPS PURPUREA)*

Ergot is a fungus that parasitizes the growing kernels of wheat and rye. Extract of ergot contains several important alkaloids, including ergometrine, which induces uterine contractions during childbirth, ergotamine, which stops bleeding and is effective against migraines if used in the early stages, and bromocriptine, which is used to treat female infertility, inhibit excessive milk production in lactating mothers, and relieve the symptoms of prostatitis and Parkinson's disease.

Caution: Ergot is highly toxic. It contains derivatives of lysergic acid, the active ingredient of LSD, which produces dangerous hallucinations and delusions. It should be used only under strict medical supervision.

ESSENTIAL FATTY ACIDS *(EFA) (VITAMIN F)* SEE FATS

EUCALYPTUS, BLUE GUM *(EUCALYPTUS GLOBULUS)*

A large, evergreen tree, native to Australia, its leaves are used to produce extracts and essential oils which are used as a disinfectant in many mouthwashes and toothpastes. Eucalyptus is also an expectorant. In addition, it can be used to soothe ulcers and to relax muscle cramps. An infusion of the fresh leaves rubbed into the scalp can help promote hair growth. Can be picked or collected. Available at larger health food stores and herbalists.

EVENING PRIMROSE *(Oenothera Biennis)*

A tall elegant annual, its spectacular yellow flowers generally open only at dusk, blooming for one night only before withering the next day. The plant was known to the ancient Greeks and flourishes throughout Europe and both North and South America. As well as being cultivated, it can frequently be found growing along roadsides.

The plant contains mucilaginous substances with sedative, diuretic and astringent properties. Infusions of all parts of the plant can be used to soothe coughs, relieve asthma, help lift depression, and also stimulate the liver and the digestive system. They can also be used to produce a soothing ointment for skin rashes. The North American Indians used the plant to treat wounds and infections externally, and coughs and colds internally.

For benefits see Evening Primrose Oil *(EPO)*.

EVENING PRIMROSE OIL *(EPO)*

The oil extracted from the seeds of the evening primrose has been found to have many beneficial effects, including: inducing weight loss without dieting; lowering cholesterol levels and blood pressure; alleviating arthritis; healing or improving eczema and acne (with zinc); and relieving premenstrual tension and irritable bowel syndrome.

EPO has also been found to be a rich source of gamma-linolenic acid (GLA). This is a fatty acid which is the starting point in the body for the production of prostaglandins (PGs), hormone-like compounds that regulate various bodily functions. Specific type of PGs perform diverse roles – and sometimes contrasting ones – and their balance is vital for health. For example, PGE1 inhibits blood clotting and increases urination, while PGE2 accelerates blood clotting and increases water retention. Deficiencies of PGs can cause many and varied conditions such as heart disease and hypertension, arthritis, menstrual cramps, allergies, asthma and migraines. Available in capsules in health food stores and pharmacies.

EXERCISE

Exercise is a nutrient that money cannot buy and, like diet, has many health benefits. Regular exercise has been found to reduce stress by releasing brain endorphins. It also strengthens the heart muscle and its activity, helps to reduce high blood pressure and high cholesterol levels, thus reducing the risk of heart attack, aids weight reduction, relieves constipation, and improves diabetes, insomnia and varicose veins. In addition, it can prevent porous bones and osteoporosis, especially in menopausal women.

Aerobic and non-aerobic exercises have different effects: aerobics involve intensive breathing and tone the heart, while non-aerobic, as in a gym workout, increase muscle tone. Exercise, like diet, should be adapted to an individual's condition and needs, preferably by a professional trainer.

F

FASTING

Fasting is one of the oldest known therapies. Nutritionally, the purpose of fasting is detoxification since purifying the body from toxins and waste substances fortifies the action of the immune system in fighting disease and promotes health and well-being. Water is a most important part of the process. At least two litres of mineral or spring water should be drunk a day to help flush out the toxins.

The immediate result of fasting is weight loss and well over a kilo (up to 3 lb.) can be lost in the first 24 hours. Fasting, however, can do much more than that. It can rejuvenate the body and help to reduce addictions to alcohol and smoking. It also releases growth hormone which strengthens immunity to disease. In various Swedish and German health clinics, fasting is used to treat virtually all degenerative diseases, from obesity, arthritis and atherosclerosis, to allergies, eczema and digestive disorders.

Long fasts or fasts intended to combat chemical poisoning should be done under medical supervision. Generally, short fasts (one to three days) do not require medical supervision.

Caution: Fasting can be dangerous for diabetics or for people with heart or kidney problems. Anyone with a health problem should seek medical clearance before fasting. A safer and easier type of fast is the 'raw juice fasting', in which small amount of freshly squeezed fruit or vegetable juices, such as apples, carrots and celery, are sipped several times a day.

FATS

One of the main food group, it is composed of fatty acids, both saturated and unsaturated. Fats are a concentrated source of energy, supplying 9 calories per gram. Hard fats are usually of animal origin, and are composed mainly of saturated fatty acids such as butter and lard. Margarine is a vegetable oil that solidifies through a process known as hydrogenation. Liquid vegetable oils, such as sunflower, safflower and corn, consist mainly of polyunsaturated omega-6 fatty acids, with the exception of palm and coconut oils, which are mostly saturated. Fish oils are also polyunsaturated, but contain omega-3 fatty acids and other beneficial factors which reduce cholesterol and the incidence of heart disease. **Olive oil** and **avocado** are monounsaturated oils. The type and structure of fatty acids determine the various types of fats – whether they are **cholesterol**, triglyceride or myelin – and different fats have different roles.

Fats are vital to the body. They enable the utilization of the fat-soluble vitamins, A, E, D and K; fats are the only substance that stimulates gall bladder activity, without which gallstones can be formed, and they are needed to produce hormones and are essential for sexual activity. Certain types of fats insulate the nerves, ensuring a healthy nerve function. Fats are also essential for skin health and beauty.

Most fatty acids can be produced in the body; the three exceptions – linoleic, linolenic and arachidonic acids (**vitamin F**) – are known as 'essential fatty acids' (EFAs) and are supplied by food. EFAs are required for the function of every cell, tissue, gland and organ. They maintain a healthy and supple skin and produce prostaglandins – hormone-like compounds that reduce blood clotting, lower hypertension and prevent heart attacks and strokes. EFAs also form red blood cells and promote immunity against disease and are essential for mental function – half of the brain is composed of EFAs.

A diet in which fat is used sparingly, mostly in the form of fresh, unrefined vegetable and marine oils, is considered beneficial in preventing heart attack and cancer.

FENNEL *(Foeniculum Vulgare)*

A perennial herb, which was originally native to the Mediterranean countries, it is now widely grown in Europe and North America. Infusions of the seeds and roots relieve flatulence, strengthen digestion, help suppress appetite and, as a result, aid weight loss. Fennel is also effective in treating colics and ulcers. The seeds and leaves are used to flavour fish dishes and the stems are used as a vegetable. Fennel is available from supermarkets and health food stores, either fresh or as a herb tea or syrup.

FENUGREEK *(Trigonella Foenumgraecum)*

An annual herb, it is one of the oldest known herbal remedies. The seeds are used as a spice and can be used to expel mucous from nasal passages. A tea made from fenugreek seeds was traditionally known to increase milk secretion in nursing mothers. Fenugreek is also used to lower blood sugar levels: in Yemenite folk medicine, it is recognized as a treatment for diabetes – a glass of water, in which a tablespoonful of fenugreek seeds has been soaked overnight, is drunk each morning. The seeds are widely available at health food stores and supermarkets.

FEVERFEW (CHRYSANTHEMUM PARTHENIUM)

A cultivated perennial herb which is native to Europe, its leaves have a strong scent when crushed and it produces clusters of small, white, daisy-like flowers in late summer. Infusions of the dried flowers are a traditional European remedy for delayed menstruation, while studies have confirmed that the crushed leaves produce a good remedy for migraine headaches. However, migraine sufferers should first verify that their problem is not caused by a food allergy. Feverfew leaves have also been reported to alleviate depression and nervous disorders. The herb is available in health food stores in capsule form.

FIBRE, DIETARY

Dietary fibre is found in many vegetable foods such as bran flakes, whole grains, beans, brown rice, psyllium seeds, fruits and vegetables. It comes in several forms, including cellulose, hemicellulose and lignin – which are insoluble in water, and pectin, gums and mucilages – which are water soluble, gel-forming fibres. Fibre adds bulk to the diet, thereby increasing stool weight and promoting bulky and speedy bowel movements.

High fibre diets are known to prevent and cure many conditions, such as constipation, hypertension, high cholesterol, heart disease, duodenal ulcers, diverticulosis, diabetes, colon cancer, haemorrhoids, irritable bowel syndrome and obesity. Dietary fibre can also reduce the feeling of hunger and contribute to weight loss. Guar gum, psyllium and oat bran are a few examples of the dietary fibre available in health food shops.

Each type of dietary fibre has its unique characteristics.

Cellulose and hemicellulose, which abound in foods such as apples, pears, whole grains and beans, are indigestible and help constipation, haemorrhoids and colitis. Lignin, which is found in foods such as whole grains, carrots, tomatoes and potatoes, is an indigestible fibre that is useful for lowering cholesterol, preventing gallstones and colon cancer. Pectin abounds in apples and is good for diabetics, lowering cholesterol and reducing the risk of heart disease and gallstones. Gums and mucilages, found in foods such as oatmeal, oatbran and beans, help to remove toxins, regulate blood sugar level and also lower cholesterol. (See also BRAN)

FIGS

The fig is considered by herbalists as a healing food. It has a detoxifying action and is one of the most alkalising fruits. That is, it balances acidic conditions in the body, which adversely affect health (see ACID-ALKALINE BALANCE). Figs are rich in mucin, which makes them a gentle laxative for treating constipation. They also soothe the digestive tract, cleanse the intestines and are helpful in the treatment of haemorrhoids. Widely available at health food stores and supermarkets.

FISH

Fish contain B vitamins, minerals like iodine, fluorine, cobalt, calcium, magnesium, phosphorus, iron and copper. Some fish like cod and haddock are virtually pure protein, having no carbohydrates and only 0.1 per cent fat. Ocean fish can also serve as protection from diseases such as atherosclerosis, heart disease, high blood pressure and cancer.

Lean fish, under 5 per cent fat, include halibut, cod, haddock, sole, flounder, perch and bass. Fatty fish − 5 to 20 per cent fat, include salmon, mackerel, herring, sardines, albacore and tuna. These fish are also a rich source of vitamins A and D.

Cold water fish, especially the fatty group, are a rich source of **omega-3 fatty acids,** which can reduce blood stickiness, high blood pressure and cholesterol levels. Fish can benefit arthritics, since its omega-3 fatty acids are also strong anti-inflammatory agents.

Fish is a rich source of iodine, known to contribute to weight loss, treating goiter and offering protection from cancer. Being high in choline, fish is known as a 'brain food'.

The hazards in fish come from water pollution. Mercury can accumulate in fish in the form of methyl mercury, which is more toxic than pure mercury. Some fresh water fish may be contaminated with industrial discharge of chemical effluents such as chlorinated hydrocarbons. See also COD LIVER OIL.

Shellfish are highly nutritious, easily digestible foods. They are high in protein, low in fat and rich in essential minerals. Except for sea clams and mussels, however, most shellfish are highly polluted. Since poisonous shellfish cannot be detected by their appearance or smell, they should be bought fresh, from reliable, uncontaminated sources.

FISH OILS

Fish oils have long been used by mothers as a food supplement for growing children. In recent years studies have shown that fish oils can also reduce the risk of coronary heart disease and lower high cholesterol levels.

The properties of fish oils first became apparent in the

investigation of Greenland Eskimos who consumed a very high-fat diet from seal, whale and fish, and yet had a low rate of heart diease. Fish oils were found to contain large amounts of omega-3 fatty acids: eicosapentaenoic acid (EPA) and docosahexaenoic acid (DHA). These are long chain and highly unsaturated fatty acids which can prevent sudden heart attacks with a variety of actions: they have an antithrombotic action which prevents thrombosis by inhibiting the formation of thromboxane A2 from arachidonic acid in platelet; they decrease blood stickiness, preventing formation of blood clots; they lower blood levels of cholesterol and triglycerides and prevent atherosclerosis; and they prevent irregular heartbeat (arrhythmia), reducing the risk of extremely rapid heart contractions (ventricular fibrillation). (See also OMEGA-3 FATTY ACIDS)

FLAXSEED (LINUM USITATISSIMUM)

Also known as linseed, this annual herb is one of mankind's oldest cultivated crops. First grown in the Middle East, and then Egypt, its cultivation spread to Western Europe in about 1000 BC and then later to North America. It is now grown worldwide for both fibre and oil production.

It is the seeds of the plant that are used for medicinal purposes. A traditional treatment for constipation is to eat 1 to 2 tablespoonfuls of ripe whole seeds, which have previously been soaked or ground, with plenty of water. The seeds swell up in the intestines and encourage bowel movement. A decoction of the seeds can be soothing to the digestive tract, and can also be used for respiratory and urinary disorders.

Linseed oil is the richest source of omega-3 fatty acids, linoleic acid and alpha-linolenic acid. These **essential fatty**

acids (**EFAs**) are vitally important for strengthening immunity and preventing many degenerative disease such as heart disease. Linseed oil is reputed to help with the elimination of gallstones – by taking a tablespoonful of the oil and then lying down for half an hour. Available at health food stores and herbalists.

FLUORINE

Fluorine is a non-metallic essential trace element which is concentrated in trace amounts in the bones and teeth. In its natural form, it occurs as calcium fluoride and sodium fluoride (used for fluoridating drinking water). Fluorine builds strong, hard bones and teeth. Its deficiency can cause tooth decay in children and fractured hips in the elderly. Tea is a good dietary source of fluorine.

Although small amounts of fluorine are important, excesses can be harmful. Excess fluorine neutralizes important enzymes, interferes with calcium absorption, creating calcium deficiencies which can cause mottled teeth, brittle bones and nervousness. Fluorinated drinking water supply should contain no more than 1 part per million (ppm), since a concentration of over 2 ppm converts fluorine from friend to foe. Brushing teeth with fluorinated toothpaste should be done carefully, to avoid swallowing the paste. Estimated adequate daily intakes are: adults 1.5–4 mg; children 1.5–2 mg.

Caution: An intake of 20 mg fluorine or over is toxic.

FOLIC ACID

Folic acid, or folacin, is one of the water–soluble B vitamins which are partly synthesized by the intestinal flora. Although its requirements are low and measured in micrograms, folic acid is a very important vitamin. Together with vitamin B12, it is crucial to the production of red blood cells, preventing anaemia, and for the synthesis of **nucleic acids** (DNA), ensuring proper cell division. It is especially critical to the development of nerves in the foetus, and a deficiency in pregnant women is linked to birth defects such as spina bifida.

However, folic acid has many other beneficial effects, in that it stimulates stomach secretions and improves digestion, increases oestrogen levels and improves lactation, promotes mental and emotional health, helps the body to produce brain neurotransmitters (chemicals which transmit messages between nerve cells), and raises histamine levels, thereby benefiting nervous disorders.

The typical Western diet is normally deficient in folic acid as it is easily destroyed in the body – its antagonists include antibiotics, contraceptive pills and anticonvulsant drugs. Pregnant and lactating women, as well as women on the pill, are particularly vulnerable to a deficiency of the vitamin and should take folic acid supplements.

The symptoms of folic acid deficiency include megaloblastic anaemia, depression, psychosis and epileptic fits, atherosclerosis, osteoporosis, acne, lack of appetite and sore tongue. Folic acid received its name from the Latin 'folium', meaning foliage, and, in fact, some of its best natural sources include green leafy vegetables such as spinach, kale and beet greens. Other sources include brewer's yeast, soya flour, wheat germ, beans, asparagus, liver, egg yolk, whole grains and avocados. The recommended daily allowance of folic acid is 200 mcg for adults, 100 mcg for children and 400 mcg for pregnant women.

Caution: Excess folic acid supplementation can mask the anaemia caused by B12 deficiency since both vitamins are closely related. These two vitamins are therefore best taken simultaneously.

FOOD ALLERGIES SEE ALLERGIES, FOOD

FOOD COMBINATION

Correct food combinations are regarded by nutritionists as the simplest and most effective way to prevent many common ailments. For instance, they are particularly beneficial to people with sensitive digestion as correct food combining has been found to prevent stomach acidity, heartburn, bloating, indigestion, constipation and headaches. It can also alleviate allergies, calm nervousness and contribute to weight loss without dieting.

The principle behind food combination is that different groups of foods require different enzymes and chemical environments for proper digestion and absorption. If, at the same meal, the body is presented with a range of ingredients each with differing requirements, it becomes confused and is not fully able to supply all the enzymes and secretions at the right time. The result can be fermentation, with all its associated discomforts.

For correct digestion, protein foods require an acid medium and proteolytic enzymes, as supplied by the stomach, while starches require an alkaline medium with starch-splitting enzymes, as supplied by the intestines. Fats and oils are digested slowly, mostly in the intestines, and do not interfere much with either protein or starch digestion.

Sugars are the quickest to digest; some are even absorbed in the stomach, while most are absorbed through the intestines.

All this means that proteins and starches make a poor combination and should not be eaten together at the same meal as they require different chemical environments and digestive processes. On the other hand, proteins and fats, or starches and fats, may be eaten together, since their digestion does not interfere with one another, but proteins should only be eaten with acid fruits, such as oranges and grape-fruits. Sweet fruits are best eaten with starches, and although sugars can be eaten with starches, they are best eaten on their own, as they are absorbed very quickly. Green vegetables and non-starchy vegetables, such as avocado, aubergine and squashes, are neutral and can be eaten with both protein or starch meals.

People with sensitive digestions may find that eating simple meals, with as few foods as possible, will alleviate their discomforts and contribute most to their well-being.

See also COMPLETE NUTRITION.

FOOD IRRADIATION

Food irradiation is used to preserve foods. Irradiation started in 1963 in the US, when permission was given to irradiate wheat and wheat flour. Its main purpose was to destroy germs and insects that spoil wheat, and inhibit ripening or sprouting. In later years, many foods were irradiated, including potatoes, spices, teas, pork, poultry, fruits and vegetables.

During irradiation, foods are exposed to extremely strong radioactive gamma rays provided by cobalt-60 or caesium-137. Although irradiation does not make the food itself radioactive, it does cause chemical changes in it, and increasing concern has been expressed on the potential hazards of irradiation. The process disrupts molecule bonds, which can recombine with other molecules, and this can produce new substances called 'radiolytic products' which pose a question of safety, since they are impossible to test. For example, some amino acids (protein) and carbohydrate groups break down and enzyme action is modified. There is also increasing evidence that irradiation destroys certain nutrients in the food such as vitamins A, B, C, E and K.

Food irradiation has been banned or severely restricted in many countries, including Britain, Germany, Denmark, Sweden, Australia and New Zealand.

FOOD PYRAMID

The Food Guide Pyramid is a guide to daily food choices which was compiled by the US Department of Agriculture (USDA) in 1992. It reflects the need for an increased consumption of vegetables, fruit grain and fibre and replaces the former dietary guidelines of the Basic Four Food Groups which promoted animal protein and fat.

The USDA has acknowledged that due to over-reliance on convenience foods, Western populations tend to be overfed but undernourished, consuming far more fat and far less fresh fruit and vegetables than is desirable. As a result, the West is plagued by the many degenerative diseases of ageing, such as heart disease, cancer and arthritis, which are scarcely found in the Asian countries with their higher consumption of fruit and vegetables.

The food pyramid contains, at its base – its widest part – the starchy group, with a recommended 6 to 11 daily servings of bread, cereal, rice and pasta. The next narrower part of the pyramid is divided into two groups: the fruit group with 2 to 4 servings, and the vegetable group with 3 to 5 servings. Next, as the pyramid narrows, it is again divided into even smaller groups: the meat, fish, eggs, beans and nut group with 2 to 3 servings, and then the milk, yogurt and cheese group with 2 to 3 servings. The small apex at the top of the pyramid signifies the group comprising fats, oils and sweets, which, it is recommended, should be used only sparingly.

Therefore, in order to meet the new USDA guidelines, one would need to eat daily, for example, one apple, one banana, one orange, four ounces of broccoli, four ounces of Brussels sprouts, four ounces of cauliflower and four ounces of spinach. Unfortunately, few of us actually eat accordingly, but we should become more conscious of the fact that it is vitally important to increase our resistance to disease by the use of the health-promoting dietary nutrients found in fresh food. Taking vitamin and mineral supplements to bridge the gap is a practical solution, but these will not replace the many auxiliary, non-vitamin nutrients contained in fresh foods.

FOOD SUPPLEMENTATION

Food supplements of vitamins, minerals, amino acids, enzymes and other nutrients are becoming increasingly popular. Supplementation serves to replace the nutrients lost in food processing, intensive farming and spraying, all of which remove nutrients from food, making it nutritionally inferior. Supplementation also corrects wrong eating habits and poor food choices, such as occasions when the diet is short of fresh fruit and vegetables, resulting in reduced intakes of nutrients. Our affluent society may be overfed, but, for the most part, it is definitely undernourished.

Another reason for food supplementation is that many people require more vitamins than others. Some burn vitamins quicker, while others may have absorption defects which create nutrient deficiencies. Stress, smoking and alcohol also deplete nutrients. However, this is only part of the answer. More people are becoming increasingly aware of their nutritional needs. The symptoms of mild nutrient deficiencies such as headaches, nervousness, fatigue, constipation, premenstrual tension and high cholesterol are no longer acceptable as part of our lot in life. More and more people want an optimal feeling of well-being, not just absence of disease – which is the medical definition of health.

FREE RADICALS SEE ANTIOXIDANTS

FRENCH PARADOX

This term describes the seemingly strange occurrence of low incidence of heart disease found in the French population, whose average diet is rich in saturated fat and alcohol. The French eat 30 per cent more fat than Americans and drink nine times more **wine**, but suffer 40 per cent fewer heart attacks. The French paradox is explained by the fact that production of red wine includes the **grape seeds**, which contain important antioxidant flavonoids, such as **quercetin**, tannins and proanthocyanidins (OPC). These ingredients of red wine have been found to provide protection from heart attacks.

FRUCTO-OLIGO SACCHARIDES *(FOS)*

These are a new class of carbohydrates, which are becoming increasingly popular in health food shops. FOS are natural sugars present in small amounts in everyday fruits, vegetables and grains, such as bananas, tomatoes, artichokes, onions, garlic, wheat and oats. They are indigestible and are not absorbed in the body as are normal sugars. Instead, they have a great beneficial effect on the intestinal flora. FOS actually feed selectively only the friendly intestinal bacteria, such as bifidobacteria and Lactobacillus acidophilus, but not the unfriendly bacteria such as Clostridium perfringens, salmonella or E. coli. In one study, a daily addition of 8 grams FOS to the diet, resulted in a ten-fold increase of the friendly bifidobacteria.

The use of FOS has far-reaching implications. By improving the intestinal flora and keeping it slightly acidic, FOS can relieve constipation, neutralize body odours and improve nutrient absorption from food.

The use of FOS is particularly important when taking antibiotics, which kill all intestinal bacteria, both friendly and unfriendly, causing conditions such as diarrhoea, yeast infections and fatigue. FOS can also benefit diabetics, reducing their levels of sugar and cholesterol.

FRUCTOSE

Fructose, also called fruit sugar, is a natural sugar present in fruits and honey. As part of the glucose molecule, it is produced from sucrose sources, such as corn. Fructose releases less insulin than sugar does over a longer period of time and is therefore used by some mild diabetics as sweetener.

G

GABA *(Gamma-aminobutyric Acid)*

An amino acid supplement (available from health food stores) which is gaining popularity for its anti-anxiety effects, GABA is produced in the body from glutamic acid and acts as an inhibitory neurotransmitter. That is, it slows down activity in the part of the brain called the lymbic system, which is our emotional alarm bell. Thus, GABA is able to help reduce stressful feelings such as anxiety, fear and panic. As a natural tranquillizer, GABA can partially replace valium by binding to the same brain receptors, providing tranquillization. It is also reported to help reduce frequent night-time urination by suppressing the hormone prolactin, which stimulates urination.

GAMMA-ORYZANOL

As an ester of ferrulic acid, gamma oryzanol is an **antioxidant** within plant cells which is widely distributed in foods such as rice, wheat, barley, oats, vegetables, olives, tomatoes and citrus fruits. Found mainly in the bran part of grains, it promotes their growth. Gamma-oryzanol was isolated from rice-bran oil and was first used by the Japanese to treat anxiety. It is now used mainly to treat the hot flushes of menopause, high cholesterol levels and digestive disorders such as ulcers, gastritis and irritable bowel syndrome.

As a potent antioxidant, gamma-oryzanol can help to prevent the damaging effects of radiation and chemotherapy. Animal studies have shown that it can also have anti-cancer effects. Many bodybuilders believe that gamma–oryzanol increases the secretion of growth hormone, since it acts on the hypothalamus and the pituitary gland, the sources of this hormone (see ARGININE). Gamma–oryzanol is considered to be a safe, natural substance and its normal total daily intake is estimated at 300 mg.

GARLIC

Garlic, a pungently flavoured bulb of the onion family, is a classic example of a combination of food and folk medicine. It contains various ingredients such as allicin, ajoene and sulphur compounds that boost the immune response and increase resistance against various diseases and which also have antibacterial, antifungal and antithrombic effects.

Garlic is extensively used to prevent and treat colds and flu. It has been found to lower blood pressure and reduce blood stickiness, thus preventing coronary thrombosis, heart attacks and strokes, and has also been found to be beneficial in inhibiting the growth of cancerous tumours, and treating diabetes, yeast infections, allergies and stress. The long–term use of garlic can benefit people who are predisposed to conditions such as heart disease, cancer or diabetes, or have a family history of them.

As a strong anti–fungal, garlic has long been a folk remedy for children with intestinal parasites such as pinworms or tapeworms. It has also been used in the treatment of athlete's foot and yeast overgrowth. For anyone concerned about the strong odour of the herb, this can be suppressed by eating fresh parsley along with it. There are also many brands of garlic oil capsules available in health food shops and, when taken in this form, no odour of garlic is left on the breath.

GENETICALLY MODIFIED FOODS *(GM)*

In recent years, genetic engineering has been applied in farming with the purpose of improving certain characteristics in plants. Genetic modification consists of splicing a gene with a desired quality from one plant and inserting it into another. In nature, only closely related plants are able to mix genes, but in genetic engineering it is possible to mix genes of entirely unrelated plants or organisms. For example, a variety of tomatoes was made frost-resistant by the insertion of an 'antifreeze' gene from an arctic fish. However, there has been concern among many people that once new genes enter the DNA chain, they can cause genetic damage with unpredictable results. For instance, in 1989, a batch of genetically engineered L-tryptophan, a calming amino acid, caused the death of 30 people in the United States and afflicted thousands of others with a rare blood disorder. This controversial subject eventually became a public issue when it became known that staple grains such as soybeans and maize, for example, were being genetically modified to resist herbicides as these grains are widely used in many human foods and also in animal feeds. Scientists became concerned that GM foods could compromise the treatment of disease in animals and humans by increasing resistance to the commonly-used antibiotic ampicillin, which could lead to the creation of drug-resistant bugs. Consumer groups and supermarkets have demanded clear labelling and the segregation of GM foods, in the hope that the GM foods of today do not become the BSE problem of tomorrow.

GERMANIUM

Germanium is a much acclaimed trace element. It is a semi-metal and semiconductor, and was once used to make transistors. Nutritionally, organic germanium boosts the immune system by stimulating the production of interferon and other immune cells, increasing resistance to various diseases. Organic germanium also lowers the oxygen requirements of body organs and is a powerful antioxidant, reducing peroxidation damage, and helping prevent the debilitating diseases of ageing. As such, it was found to have a beneficial effect on ovarian malignancies, colon cancer and Hodgkin's disease. Organic germanium was also found to have anti-arthritic properties.

Trace amounts of germanium are present in most foods, but richer amounts are found in ginseng, garlic, aloe vera and comfrey, which may partially explain the health-promoting effects of these foods. Germanium is also available as a supplement at health food stores.

GINKGO BILOBA

A tree which is thought to have existed for over 200 million years, its leaves were recently found to contain substances capable of reversing the ageing of the brain. Strong antioxidant flavones, which make up 47 per cent of ginkgo extract, are considered to halt lipid peroxidation in the brain and protect the membranes of brain cells.

Since ginkgo appears to increase both blood supply and oxygen supply to the brain, it is possible that it could benefit sufferers of degenerative diseases such as dementia in the elderly, which is considered to be a result of poor flow of blood and oxygen to the brain. Indeed, studies have shown that ginkgo biloba extracts can benefit senility and sufferers of Alzheimer's disease, and also help to improve short-term memory loss.

Ginkgo biloba extract capsules are available in health food stores. It is recommended that a minimum usage period of three months is necessary to achieve any benefit.

GINGER *(ZINGIBER OFFICINALIS)*

A perennial plant which is grown in most of the tropical regions of the world, its powdered root has been used for centuries as a culinary spice and in infusions. Ginger is a stimulant that relieves flatulence, discharges mucous, strengthens digestion, stimulates glandular secretions and relieves vomiting. Blended with cinnamon powder, ginger makes a pleasant tea and ginger root powder taken in doses of 250 mg four times a day can effectively reduce early pregnancy nausea. In some African cultures, ginger is considered to be an aphrodisiac.

GINSENG *(PANAX GINSENG)*

Ginseng is the most widely used herb of Chinese medicine, hence its name, *panax*, which means 'cure-all'. It is a small perennial plant, native to Korea, but also cultivated in China, Siberia and the US. Ginseng is grown for its root which is said to abound with healing properties and which is used mainly as a tonic. Its many uses, however, include treatment for a great variety of disorders, from hypertension, fatigue and stress, to weak memory, arthritis and impotence. The root contains glycosides, called ginsenosides, with vitamins and minerals which fortify the immune system, increasing resistance to various diseases, and promoting physical and mental vigour. Ginseng is available from health food shops as teas, capsules and extracts.

GLANDULAR THERAPY

Eating raw animal glands, such as the liver, is a practice which has been followed since ancient times to invigorate the body and fight disease. The therapeutic value of endocrine glands, which secrete hormones and enzymes, has recently been gaining increased scientific recognition, and following the development of safe production methods, such as freeze-drying, which preserve the nutrients of the glands, glandular supplements have become available.

The principle underlying glandular therapy is that 'like cures like'. For example, a person with a weak liver or liver disease can benefit by eating animal liver. Indeed, science has confirmed that glandular extracts of various glands such as those of the thyroid, adrenal, thymus, pancreas or pituitary, are quite effective when taken orally because of their active hormone and enzyme content. **Pancreatin**, for example, is a popular digestive aid made from the pancreas gland, which contains a comprehensive range of digestive enzymes. The adrenal gland is rich in hormones and its extracts are used to overcome stress and many other ailments, such as asthma, heart disease, flu, depression, headaches, irritable bowel syndrome, diabetes, PMS and arthritis.

Glandular extracts are now available in health food shops in various combinations, on their own, and included in multivitamin preparations.

GLAZING AGENTS

These are food additives, such as beeswax or shellac, which are used by the food industry to give foods a shiny appearance or a protective coating.

GLA see EVENING PRIMROSE OIL *(EPO)*

GLUCOMANNAN

A gum, which is derived from a plant tuber, it acts as dietary fibre by absorbing water and, in the intestines, can expand to 60 times its weight. It is also a fat mobilizer, combining with fat to removes it from the colon. Thus, glucomannan can be used to treat constipation, curb appetite, normalize blood sugar levels, help with weight loss, reduce cholesterol levels and treat diabetes.

Glucomannan is sold in capsules, and for best results, two to three capsules should be taken with a large glass of water half an hour before meals.

GLUCONATES

These are mineral complexes bound with gluconic acid. Gluconic acid is naturally produced by the body and used as a source of energy. The gluconate complex enables minerals to cross the intestinal wall and be absorbed into the blood stream more efficiently. Mineral gluconates, sold in health food shops, include iron, zinc, calcium, magnesium, potassium, manganese and copper. (See CHELATION)

GLUCOSE TOLERANCE FACTOR *(GTF)* SEE CHROMIUM

GLUCOSE

Also known as blood sugar, it is the form of sugar which is produced in plant and animal tissues and used to provide energy. It is the end product of assimilated foods, and a feeling of well-being and high energy levels depend upon the maintenance of normal levels of glucose in the blood, cells and muscles. The brain is particularly dependent on glucose as its energy source: a drop in the brain's glucose level immediately releases hormones, such as adrenaline and glucagone, to restore it. A chronic condition of low blood glucose levels is known as hypoglycaemia, while its opposite – chronic high glucose levels – is diabetes. Glucose is found naturally in fruits, grains and plants.

GLUCOSE TOLERANCE TEST *(GTT)*

This is standard laboratory test for detecting hypoglycaemia or diabetes. To check for diabetes, the patient is normally given a solution of 100 grams glucose to drink first thing in the morning, on an empty stomach, and blood samples are then taken after 30 minutes, and again after an hour, to check the glucose levels. The most reliable GTT for hypoglycaemia is one that lasts for five to six hours, with blood samples being taken each hour.

GLUCOSAMINE SULPHATE *(GS)*

Glucosamine sulphate is a compound which occurs naturally in the joints. It is made up of glucose, an amino acid (glutamine) and sulphur. Its main function is to stimulate the growth of cartilage, by serving as a building block for its production. GS provides proteoglycans (PAS), protein and sugar molecules that attract and hold water, and produces a group of gelatinous compounds known as glycosaminoglycans (GAGs), which bind water in the cartilage matrix and help prevent cartilage from breaking down. GS also promotes the incorporation of sulphur into the cartilage, which means that GS is not only necessary for joint function, but also for stimulating its repair. In this sense, GS works best with chondroitin sulphate (CS) to repair cartilage damage, preventing osteoarthritis. While GS holds water in the cartilage, CS acts more like a "water magnet".

In many people, the production of GS in the body declines with age, as cartilage loses its flexibility as a shock absorber and the result is osteoarthritis, the most common form of arthritis, which affects millions of elderly people. It has been suggested that GS deficiency is the major causative factor in osteoarthritis and, as a result, GS supplements have been tried and found successful in the treatment of the disease.

GS is now widely available in health food stores as a dietary supplement.

Taken orally, it is efficiently absorbed and tolerated with no known contra-indications or adverse interactions with drugs. In some cases of nausea or heartburn, it is advised that GS should be taken with meals. The standard dose is 500 mg, three times a day, but overweight people may require more, depending on their body weight (20 mg per kg of body weight a day).

GLUTAMINE and GLUTAMIC ACID

Glutamic acid is a non–essential amino acid which has been described as 'brain fuel'. It is usually supplied by food and is the most prominent amino acid in wheat. Glutamic acid combines with poisonous ammonia in the brain and detoxifies it, producing glutamine, the actual brain booster. Glutamine improves brain function, alertness and mood, and can help in the treatment of alcoholism and migraines, and also to overcome a sweet tooth. Glutamic acid, by helping produce **GABA** (a calming neurotransmitter) in the body, has an indirect calming effect. However, glutamine is better absorbed than glutamic acid and is available as a supplemental amino acid in health food shops.

GLUTATHIONE, L-GLUTATHIONE

A potent antioxidant, it is a peptide produced in the body from three amino acids, glycine, glutamic and cysteine. Glutathione helps to prevent many of the degenerative diseases of ageing, such as heart disease, cancer and arthritis, and it is also thought to increase life-span. This is a result of its participation in various enzyme systems such as glutathione peroxidase and glutathione reductase, that neutralize free radicals and reduce their oxidative damage. Since glutathione is abundant in the lens, it is especially helpful in preventing the progression of eye cataracts. It also provides protection from the effects of pollution, smoking and radiation and is a detoxifier of toxic metals and drugs. Its levels in the body can be raised by increasing intake of its precursor amino acids, glycine, glutamic and cysteine. Glutathione is available as a food supplement from health food shops.

GLUTEN

This is the major wheat protein, containing sub-divisions such as gliadins and glutenins. Gluten is high in the amino acids glutamine and proline, but low in lysine. It is also found in rye, oats, barley and buckwheat.

Gluten is the main allergy-causing ingredient in bread, and the allergy can be manifested in a variety of symptoms. An intolerance to gluten is the cause of coeliac disease, which is an intestinal malabsorption syndrome, characterized by diarrhoea, weight loss, bleeding tendency and low calcium levels. The only treatment for coeliac disease is the maintenance of a strict gluten-free diet; this is usually high in rice and maize, and should be devised by a dietician or nutritionist. Food labels must be read carefully to avoid coeliac-causing ingredients. Recent reports also implicate gluten in gastrointestinal disorders in people with sensitive digestion, and it is also suspected to be a causative factor in schizophrenia.

GLYCINE

A non-essential amino acid which, as an inhibitory neurotransmitter, inhibits stress response in the spinal cord and, together with taurine, helps to relieve spasms and contractions that are due to stress or anxiety. Glycine promotes muscle tone by increasing **creatine**, a source of high energy phosphate released during muscle contraction, and its inhibitory action contributes to the prevention of epilepsy. Glycine is also reported to reduce uric acid levels, thus benefiting gout, and it is involved in the production of glutathione, the important antioxidant enzyme.

GOLDENSEAL *(HYDRASTIS CANADENSIS)*

A small perennial herb, native to North America, it is cultivated for its medicinal uses. It has a wide range of therapeutic properties which are attributed to its high content of
active alkaloids, such as berberine, hydrastine and canadine.
It was traditionally used by the American Indians to treat a
variety of conditions, especially infections. More recently, it
has been well-documented as an antibiotic and a booster of
the body's immune system, thus useful in fighting diseases.
Goldenseal is also known as an antiseptic, diuretic and tonic.

An infusion of goldenseal can be used as a vaginal
douche and as an antiseptic mouthwash. It is also particularly
helpful in treating mucous membranes, making it useful for
colds and catarrhal conditions. Goldenseal is available from
health food stores on its own in powder, tinctures and
extracts and is increasingly included in many nutritional
formulas.

Caution: The herb must not be eaten fresh as it can
produce ulceration of the digestive tract.

GOTU-KOLA *(HYDROCOTYLE ASIATICA, CENTELLA ASIATICA)*

A native of India and Asia, gotu-kola is a mildly bitter herb
that stimulates the central nervous system. It contains several
active ingredients, such as saponins and triterpenes, which
are known to improve memory and learning ability and, in
addition, the herb is now being used to alleviate fatigue and
depression, increase sex drive, treat rheumatism, increase urination, treat heart conditions and accelerate the healing of
wounds. In Europe, gotu-kola is used to promote the self-
healing of skin ulcerations or bedsores from prolonged con-
finement to bed. In addition, in combination with cayenne

and ginger, gotu-kola has been found to be an effective energy booster. This combination can be found in health food shops under different brand names, while gotu-kola is available on its own in capsules containing the powdered herb.

GRAINS

Grains are a primary nutritional source of complex **carbohydrates**, which are mainly starch. Whole grains, and their products, also contain large amounts of fibre, vitamins and minerals, and as such are valuable as a nutritious source of energy. This food category includes wheat, barley, buckwheat, corn, rice, millet, oats, rye, triticale, amaranth and kamut.

GRAPEFRUIT

A citrus fruit, which is rich in vitamins A and C, the grapefruit contains smaller amounts of minerals such as calcium, phosphorus and potassium. The grapefruit comes both in white and pink varieties, but the pink variety has over five times the amount of vitamin A as its white counterpart. Juice from fresh grapefruits harvested in September – October is the richest in vitamin C, and is beneficial in colds and fevers.

The grapefruit peel (rind) which is rich in bioflavonoids, has a pungent, bitter-sweet flavour. The bioflavonoid activity of the peel, combined with its vitamin C content, is useful in strengthening weak gums, arteries and capillaries. To extract the properties of the peel, a tea can be prepared by simmering fresh or dried peel for twenty minutes. Externally, a compress of this tea can be used to treat frostbite by helping to restore circulation to the damaged tissue. The bitter seeds of the grapefruit are known to be a natural antibiotic.

GRAPES

Grapes contain valuable cell salts which are known to purify the blood and cleanse the body from toxins, thus benefiting kidneys and liver, and strengthening the immune response. They traditionally treat conditions such as arthritis. Grapes are diuretic, reduce water retention (oedema) and treat urinary problems; the dark varieties are beneficial in the treatment of anaemia. Grape juice can be helpful for liver conditions such as hepatitis and jaundice. The so-called 'grape cure' is a form of fasting, normally lasting between a week and ten days, during which only grapes and grape juice are consumed. Proponents of this therapy claim that, by its purifying effects, this regime is very beneficial to a wide variety of conditions as it rejuvenates the body and fortifies the immune system.

GRAPE SEEDS

Grape seeds are one of the richest sources of the plant flavonoids known as OPCs (oligomeric proanthocyanidins). These OPCs are the precursors of anthocyanins, which are the reddish-purple colouring in the skin of grapes. OPCs are potent antioxidants and, as such, have been found to be 20 times more effective than vitamin C. Studies of OPCs have revealed their effectiveness in treating circulatory disorders by strengthening the capillaries, reducing hypertension and the risk of heart attack. Grape seed extracts are available in capsules which are normally marketed as OPCs. Grape seed oil is also available for kitchen use. (See also FRENCH PARADOX)

GREEN TEA *(Camellia Sinensis)*

Green tea is produced from the same plant as the common black tea which is usually consumed in Western countries. However, it is not processed, as is the case with black tea, nor is it allowed to ferment after harvesting and before drying, and so it retains most of its active ingredients.

As a result of some studies made largely in the 1990s, green tea has been found to have many beneficial effects. It contains large amounts of catechins, a group of antioxidant substances with strong anti-cancer properties, and the tea has also been found to provide protection against oesophageal cancer and to block the formation of tumours arising in the skin, lung, digestive tract, liver and breasts. In addition, it was found to reduce cholesterol levels and lower blood pressure, and it has been claimed to fight colds and flu, prevent gum disease, dental cavities and bad breath.

Green tea bags are available in health food shops. It is recommended that three to five cups of the tea are drunk each day in order to reap its full benefits.

GROWTH HORMONE *(GH)*

This hormone is secreted by the pituitary gland in the brain and is crucial for the growth and repair of body cells, as well as for stimulating the immune system. It is secreted mainly during the first 90 minutes of night sleep, and also in response to fasting and non-aerobic, peak-effort exercise. It

is abundant in young people up to 30 years of age, and absent, or present only in small amounts, in older and/or obese people. GH has many important functions: it stimulates the growth of immune cells and is well-known to benefit auto-immune diseases such as arthritis; it speeds the healing of wounds; it stimulates muscle growth and increases the burning of fat to energy, aiding weight loss.
Supplements of several nutrients, taken on an empty stomach, can increase the release of GH in older people. GH releasers include the amino acids arginine, ornithine and the prescription drug L-Dopa (see ARGININE).

Caution: GH releasers should not be used by young persons who have not completed their growth or reached their full height.

GUARANA *(Paulinia Cubana)*

A tall climbing vine, native to the Brazilian Amazon, the seeds or beans of guarana are roasted and ground for use as a beverage in Latin America. Prepared in a similar way to coffee, guarana is high in stimulating alkaloids such as caffeine, saponins, tannins and guaranine. It is a very stimulating beverage that is claimed to relieve headaches and migraines rather quickly. Guarana also inhibits appetite and it is used as an appetite-suppressant ingredient in various slimming products. It is also used to treat arthritis and to stimulate a delayed menstruation, and is reputed to be an effective sexual stimulant. It is available in a variety of forms, including tablets and as drinks.

GUAR GUM (*CYAMOPSIS TETRAGONOLOBUS*)

Originally grown in India as a herb for livestock feed, guar gum is now used both as a food additive and as a health-promoting nutrient. It contains mucilaginous substances which are gel and bulk forming and is used in the food industry as a stabilizer and thickening agent (E412) in the production of products such as soups, salad dressings, ice cream and tooth pastes.

Nutritionally, guar gum can contribute to weight loss. It benefits slimmers by acting as a bulking agent in the digestive tract. This delays stomach emptying and the passage of food through the intestines, promoting a feeling of fullness and reducing food cravings. The gel-forming guar gum also combines with fats and promotes their excretion. Thus, it can effectively lower high cholesterol levels. Guar gum also reduces insulin levels and is beneficial for diabetics. It is available in health food stores in capsule form.

GUMS, PLANT

Plant gums are mucilaginous resins produced by various plants, usually as a response to injury. Commercially, they are produced by making a scratch in a plant or tree and collecting the exuding thick fluid. Plant gums are water-soluble and gel-forming and are used mainly by the food industry as emulsifiers and stabilizers. Examples of these are gum arabic (E414) used in confectionery and karaya gum (E416) used in soft cheeses and brown sauces.

H

HAWTHORN *(CRATAEGUS MONOGYNA)*

A European shrub, its flowers and berries contain many active flavonoid compounds. Infusions, or a few drops of tincture, are widely used in Europe in the treatment of heart disorders (particularly those of nervous origin), insomnia and hypertension. Extracts of hawthorn dilate and relax coronary vessels, reducing blood pressure and improving blood supply to the heart, and are therefore beneficial in the prevention and treatment of angina pectoris. The reddish-blue colouring of hawthorn berries is a pigment rich in anthocyanidins and proanthocyanidins. These flavonoids are potent antioxidants; they also stabilize cell membranes and fight infections. (See also GRAPES; BIOFLAVONOIDS) Available at health food stores and incorporated in formulas.

HDL *(HIGH DENSITY LIPOPROTEINS)*

A beneficial, 'friendly' form of cholesterol carrier which transports **cholesterol** to the liver for metabolism and excretion from the body. Thus, HDL prevents the build up of cholesterol deposits in the arteries, which is the cause of atherosclerosis and heart disease.

HEMICELLULOSE

Hemicellulose is an indigestible fibre that absorbs water and expands in the digestive tract. It promotes bowel movements and can help to prevent constipation and promote weight loss. It is also useful in the prevention of colon cancer by its action in reducing cancer-causing compounds in the digestive tract. One of its chief sources is oat bran, but it is also found in other whole grains, fruits and vegetables, such as apples, bananas, pears, beans, corn and peppers.

HESPERIDINE SEE BIOFLAVONOIDS

HISTIDINE

A non-essential amino acid that is found abundantly in cereals, many people are deficient in histidine. It is a precursor of histamine, which stimulates cell growth and reproduction and is very versatile in its actions, from promoting wound healing to stimulating hair growth. As a histamine precursor, histidine has a relaxing effect and can help calm anxiety feelings. It also increases gastric juices and thus prevents indigestion and ulcers. Histidine can also dispel frigidity in women and, in sufficient quantities, intensify orgasm. Available at health food stores as a supplement.

HMB (BETA-HYDROXY-BETA-METHYLBUTYRATE)

HMB is an exciting new food supplement which has been found to improve both health and appearance. It is not a steroid or a drug, but a natural chemical which is made in the body as a metabolite of the essential amino acid **leucine**. It is also present in small amounts in both vegetable and animal foods. HMB is a natural component of mother's milk, which underlines its nutritive role. Recent studies have shown that HMB helps to strengthen the immune system, lower high cholesterol levels, counteract stress and build strong muscles. In addition, studies with bodybuilders have shown that HMB can increase gains in muscle size and strength by up to 50 per cent. It has also been found to contribute to weight loss. In several studies, HMB has been shown to reduce body fat and promote leaner body mass. One researcher has commented that it seems as though 'HMB helps melt body fat'.

It is estimated that between one quarter of a gram to one gram of HMB is produced daily by the body, depending on the protein intake. Alfalfa and some fish are among the richest sources. Daily supplements of one to two grams are considered normal to obtain reasonable results, and three grams a day are recommended for athletes on intensive programmes. Since it is a component of breast milk, HMB is considered to be a safe supplement.

HONEY

Raw unheated honey is a good substitute for sugar and, in fact, is sweeter than sugar and is absorbed more quickly. The colour and flavour of honey vary according to the origin of its flowers and nectar. The sweetness of honey is a combination of simple sugars: glucose, fructose, maltose and sucrose. In addition to its sugar content, it contains the B vitamins, some minerals and enzymes, and it does not upset the mineral balance as refined sugar does. Honey has been used therapeutically for centuries, traditionally to treat sore throats and coughs, stomach ulcers, canker sores of the mouth and lips, high blood pressure and constipation. It also has a harmonizing and calming effect. Externally, it can be applied to wounds and burns.

HOP *(Humulus Lupulus)*

A perennial climbing vine found wild, it is cultivated mainly for its flowers which are used in beer making. These secrete lupulin which gives beer its bitterness and aroma. Hops are a mild diuretic and have a strong sedative action. Infusions of the dried herb have a calming effect on the nervous system and are good for stress, restlessness and insomnia. A tea prepared from hops will improve the appetite, strengthen digestion, cleanse the blood, stimulate bile secretion, and is also said to eliminate intestinal worms. Usually, no more than one cup of the tea or infusion per day is recommended. They are also available in some health food stores in capsule form.

Caution: It is important not to exceed the dosage on the label of the capsules.

Hops are available at grocers.

HORSE CHESTNUT *(Aesculus Hippocastanum)*

A tall deciduous tree, which is native to Asia, Europe and North America, it is also commonly cultivated. An infusion of the bark is good for diarrhoea, and an infusion of the fruit is beneficial in the relief of bronchitis. The seeds, which grow in large leathery capsules, contain aescin and have long been used traditionally to treat varicose veins and haemorrhoids. Aescin has anti-oedema and anti-inflammatory properties. New studies done with aescin taken orally have confirmed its ability to assist in the treatment of varicose veins and thrombophlebitis. Externally, aescin can help with the treatment of bruises.

Caution: Aescin is a mild toxin. The seeds and capsules of horse chestnut, which contain aescin, can cause poisoning if taken in sufficient amounts. Roasting the seeds seems to render the toxin harmless.

HORSETAIL (*EQUISETUM ARVENSE*)

A tall herb with a cane-like appearance, it is found wild in Europe and is also cultivated. Horsetail leaves are one of the richest sources of silica and can be used as an ingredient in silica supplements. As such, horsetail can increase calcium absorption, strengthen bones, teeth and hair, and promote a healthy and good-looking skin. Horsetail also contains other minerals such as calcium, copper and zinc, and is used as a diuretic and in the treatment of kidney stones. Horsetail is available in tablets and capsules.

HYSSOP (*HYSSOPUS OFFICINALIS*)

Hyssop's leaves are astringent and can be used to relieve flatulence and stimulate menstruation. Infusions of the leaves are also used to improve digestion, suppress coughs and relieve intestinal congestion. Decoctions are said to relieve inflammations. Available at health food stores and herbalists.

Caution: Do not use for periods of longer than a few weeks.

I

ICELAND MOSS *(Cebtraria Islandica)*

This is a small branched lichen found wild in cool damp places in the northern hemisphere. Iceland moss tea is used for bronchitis and coughs, for strengthening digestion and relieving digestive disorders. It can also help to stimulate milk flow in nursing mothers. The plant itself is nourishing and can be eaten as a vegetable after being boiled for a while to make it palatable. Available at health food stores and herbalists.

Caution: Prolonged use can cause liver or intestinal problems.

INOSITOL

Inositol is a lipotropic B vitamin, thus helping to metabolize fats and cholesterol. It combines with phosphorus, fatty acids and nitrogen to form phospholipids, which carry fat and form cell membranes. With choline, it forms lecithin. Inositol is concentrated in the brain, and supplements produce a calming effect. In cereals, seeds and legumes, inositol occurs as phytic acid, which binds with calcium, iron, zinc and other minerals, inhibiting their absorption. To prevent this, cereals and legumes which contain phytic acid, must be cooked, leavened or sprouted.

Inositol can help to lower cholesterol levels, maintain a healthy skin and lower high oestrogen levels, which can lead to breast lumps. Inositol, which is best taken at bedtime, can, in daily doses of 2,000 mg, lower high blood pressure and induce sleep. It also has an anti-anxiety effect.

The best natural sources of inositol are organ meats, brewer's yeast, wheat germ, cantaloupe, molasses and peanut butter. A recommended daily allowance has not yet been established, but a daily consumption of 1,000 mg is advised by many nutritionists.

Available at health food stores.

INVERT SUGAR

Invert sugar is obtained by breaking down sucrose into its components, glucose and fructose. This is done chemically and enzymatically. Invert sugar is a liquid sweetener, sweeter than white sugar and is sometimes used as a processed food ingredient. It is naturally contained in honey and fruits and it is less taxing on the digestive system than normal sugar (sucrose).

IODINE

An essential trace element, iodine is a constituent of the hormone thyroxine, concentrated in the thyroid gland. As with all trace elements, a tiny amount has an enormous effect on our health. An average human body contains 25 mg iodine.

The influence of iodine, through thyroxine, is felt everywhere in the body. It raises the metabolic rate, helping the body to burn excess fat, preventing the accumulation of cholesterol and helping to stabilize body weight. Iodine calms nerves and improves the quality of hair, skin, nails, and teeth.

It also regulates the rate at which cells use oxygen, and in this way promotes energy production and improves mental function. It accomplishes all this by stimulating the thyroid gland to produce thyroxine. A properly functioning thyroid is of extreme importance. An underactive thyroid, resulting from iodine deficiency, can cause symptoms such as obesity, rapid pulse, goitre, a cold body, constipation, general weakness, excessive menstruation, low resistance to colds and infections, nervousness and irritability. Iodine deficiency can also increase the risk of breast and uterine cancer.

A study of Japanese women, who normally eat plenty of seafood, which is rich in iodine, has shown that their diet contributed to their lower-than-average incidence of breast cancer.

In cases of underactive thyroid, or when taking iodine supplements, raw vegetables of the brassica family (broccoli, Brussels sprouts, cabbage, kale, cauliflower, turnip) should not be eaten. They contain a factor which inhibits the absorption of iodine. People living in areas where the soil has a low iodine content, such as the American Midwest, are prone to iodine deficiency and should take iodine supplements or eat an iodine-rich diet.

Some of the best natural sources of iodine are kelp, seaweeds, shellfish and onions. Available supplements include iodized salt, kelp tablets, dried seaweeds and desiccated bovine thyroid tablets or capsules. The normal daily requirement is 150 mcg for adults and 120 mcg for children.

IRON

Iron is the most abundant trace element in the body. The average adult body contains about 5 g, bound with protein. Iron is indispensable for the production of haemoglobin, the red pigment in red blood cells, which transports oxygen to every cell. Without iron, the body cells would 'suffocate' and die. It promotes energy, relieves fatigue, prevents anaemia and increases resistance to disease.

However, iron absorption can be problematic. Only about 8 per cent of ingested iron is actually absorbed and assimilated; for proper absorption, iron needs adequate stomach acid, a deficiency of which is common in the elderly, while protein, copper, calcium and vitamins C, B6, B12 and E are also needed for optimal iron absorption. The most easily assimilated forms of iron are the organic ones such as ferrous succinate or gluconate. Inorganic iron, such as ferrous sulphate, actually destroys vitamin E. Natural iron syrups and iron-fed brewer's yeast, which are widely available in health food stores, are also well absorbed.

Small losses of iron are normal: men lose about 1 mg a day and women lose much more, due to menstruation or pregnancy. Women, children and the elderly are more vulnerable to iron deficiency: studies have found that about a quarter of British children under five are seriously deficient in iron. Among the best natural sources of iron are liver, raw clams and oysters, oatmeal, prunes, egg yolks, brewer's yeast and green leafy vegetables.

Recommended daily dosages for iron are estimated at 10 mg for men and 18 mg for women, but requirements increase during pregnancy, lactation, and in any bleeding conditions such as excessive menstruation, ulcers or intestinal bleeding. Excess consumption of coffee and tea can cause a depletion of iron.

ISOLEUCINE

Isoleucine is one of the essential amino acids. It also one of the three branched chain amino acids, and as such is used by the muscles. Together with leucine and valine, isoleucine builds up muscle, helps to repair muscle injuries and combats stress. Isoleucine is needed for haemoglobin (blood) formation and for the regulation of blood sugar levels. Natural sources of isoleucine include legumes such as soybeans. As a supplement, isoleucine is sold as a free amino acid, but it is normally combined in a formula with **leucine** and **valine**, the other two branched chain amino acids.

J

JASMINE (*JASMINUM OFFICINALIS*)

A vine with both deciduous and evergreen varieties, it was originally native to the warm regions of the eastern hemisphere. The plant is now widely cultivated in Europe and North America, mainly for its sweet-smelling white flowers which have medicinal properties. Jasmine tea (widely available in supermarkets and health food stores), which is highly scented, has a calming effect on the nerves and can also stimulate perspiration and help to reduce fever.

JUNIPER (*JUNIPERUS COMMUNIS*)

An evergreen shrub or small tree, it grows throughout the northern hemisphere in countries with a cold climate. Juniper berries are so rich in natural sugars that they are used in the fermentation of gin, which partly retains the flavour of juniper oil. The berries, which are also used in cooking to add flavour, or made into infusions, can stimulate the appetite. They contain bitter principles, which stimulate gastric acid secretion and improve digestion, and terpenes (essential oils), which are antiseptic and help to alleviate respiratory diseases and expel phlegm from lungs. Juniper berries are also beneficial for digestive tract infections and cramps.

Caution: Juniper is not recommended for people with kidney problems.

K

KALE

An ancient member of the **brassica** family, kale is a very
nutritious green vegetable. It is a rich source of vitamins A,
B1, B2, C and niacin, as well as chlorophyll and many minerals, such as calcium, magnesium, iron, sulphur, sodium and
potassium. The juice of kale can be used to treat stomach
and duodenal ulcers, while the leaves and stalks, when eaten
as a vegetable, provide a rich source of roughage.

KAVA-KAVA *(PIPER METHYSTICUM)*

A perennial shrub, it is native to Polynesia and other Pacific
islands, where its roots and rhizomes were produced as
drinks that were traditionally used both as a folk medicine
and for ceremonial purposes. Nowadays, kava is used to alleviate anxiety, tension and restlessness. Since its rhizomes
contain kava lactones, active ingredients which promote
relaxation without loss of mental sharpness, this makes it
very useful for the daytime management of anxiety. In addition to its relaxation properties, kava is reported to increase
mental acuity, improve memory, promote restful sleep and
reduce pain.

Kava is now available from health food shops in tea bags
and capsule form. A normal daily dose is 100 mg and a
usage period of four weeks is recommended for its anti-
anxiety action to be effective.

Caution: Kava-kava is not recommended for pregnant or lactating women. Its only reported side-effect is a mild gastrointestinal disturbance, but prolonged use may cause a temporary skin yellowing. This indicates that its use should be discontinued as overdosages can lead to skin rash.

KELP

Kelp includes any of a variety of large brown seaweeds which are found in cold waters throughout the world, growing underwater and on rocky shores; it does not grow in tropical waters. In many countries, kelp is harvested from the ocean to be used as a food, or dried and sold in powder, tablet or capsule form. Kelp contains an abundance of minerals and trace elements, but it is mainly valued for being one of the richest sources of **iodine**: fresh kelp contains about 100,000 mcg iodine per pound, while dried kelp contains nearly ten times as much.

In addition to iodine, kelp also contains carbohydrates, both in the form of sugar and starches. Its sugar is **mannitol**, which is not very sweet and is a mild laxative. As mannitol does not raise blood sugar levels, it is excellent for use by diabetics. Kelp also contains small amounts of vitamins A, B and C, and a substance, sodium alginate, which binds with radioactive strontium-90, preventing its absorption and promoting its excretion from the body. Thus, kelp can provide protection from radioactive fallout. Through its high iodine content, it can also reduce the risk of cancer. The high iodine diet of the Japanese, who eat plenty of seaweeds, has been linked to the low incidence of breast cancer in Japan.

Caution: people with an overactive thyroid, pregnant or lactating women, should consult a doctor before using kelp.

KOHLRABI

A green vegetable of the **Brassica** family, it is grown for its large, edible stem which has a slight sweetish–bitter flavour similar to turnip. Kohlrabi can improve blood circulation, strengthen digestion and help to stabilize blood sugar levels, making it beneficial for diabetics and hypoglycaemics. It can also help to relieve painful urination, stop internal bleeding, and purify the body from toxins and alcohol. The juice is considered a remedy for nosebleeds.

KOLA, KOLA NUT *(COLA VERA)*

The kola is a large tree which grows wild in West Africa and is also cultivated in South America. The kola nut contains caffeine and is well known as a nerve stimulant. It fights fatigue and promotes strength and endurance and is also used as a heart tonic. Kola nut is used in the production of some of the popular soft drinks.

KOMBU

Kombu is a seaweed related to **kelp**. It contains a number of minerals and is especially high in **iodine**. It is usually available from health food stores as dried leaves which can be added to soups and stews. Because of its high mineral content, kombu greatly enhances the nutritional value of any foods prepared with it. It is especially useful when added to beans and legumes as it increases their digestibility. As with any high-iodine food, it improves thyroid function and can help in treating all conditions resulting from iodine deficiency.

KOMBUCHA

A recently rediscovered 'mushroom', which has been known and used for centuries in Asian countries, kombucha tea is being increasingly acclaimed in the West for its great healing benefits.

Although it appears to be a mushroom, kombucha is in fact a colony of yeast and bacteria. It grows and propagates in a solution of weak tea and sugar which, as the kombucha grows, begins to ferment, producing carbon dioxide and alcohol. When the kombucha has doubled in size, it is removed from the solution to start a new batch. The resulting liquid, which is biologically active, is kept refrigerated, to be drunk daily in six-ounce doses.

The tea has antibiotic, antibacterial and antiviral properties and purifies the body by binding to toxins and promoting their excretion. It contains several of the B vitamins and glucuronic acid, a known liver detoxifier. Kombucha cleanses the liver and kidneys, creating several health benefits such as increasing energy, strengthening digestion and skin improvement. Although these benefits may vary in individuals, people have reported amazing improvements in a range of chronic conditions, from psoriasis, constipation and fatigue to thyroid deficiency, hair fall and brittle nails.

Ready-made kombucha tea is now available in many health food shops in bottles and as extract drops.

Caution: Kombucha tea is not recommended for diabetics.

KUDZU *(Radix Puerariae)*

A Chinese herb, kudzu is a fast-growing vine which is native to the Orient and was introduced into the United States during the latter part of the nineteenth century.

Although it is known in the southern United States as a nuisance weed, kudzu has long been used in traditional Chinese medicine for the management of alcohol abuse. A recent study carried out by Harvard University proved its ability to reduce alcohol intake in hamsters. When given kudzu extract, the animals seem to prefer water over alcohol. Two isoflavone compounds in kudzu, daidzein and daidzin, were identified as being responsible for the anti-alcohol effect. The herb is now marketed by some US vitamin manufacturers.

L

LACTOBACILLUS

This is the comprehensive name for a group of bacteria in the intestines. They are non-motile, do not produce spores and are acid resistant. They convert carbohydrates to lactic acid in the intestines, and are used to sour milk and make yogurts. The family of Lactobacillus include, for example, Lactobacillus Acidophilus and Lactobacillus Bulgaricus. (See also PROBIOTICS)

LACTOSE, LACTOSE INTOLERANCE

Lactose is milk sugar obtained from the evaporation of cow's milk. As a disaccharide, it is made up of glucose and galactose. In the souring of milk (as in the production of yogurt), lactose is converted to lactic acid. The milk of mammals contains between 4 to 7 per cent lactose, which cannot be absorbed as such. To absorb lactose, newborns have to secrete the enzyme lactase which breaks down lactose to its components, glucose and galactose, which are absorbable. However, after weaning and growing to adulthood, many people lose their ability to secrete lactase and cannot therefore digest milk or dairy products. This condition is known as 'lactose intolerance' and affects some 70 to 90 per cent of oriental, black, native American and Mediterranean adults, whereas the rate among northern and western Europeans is as low as 15 per cent.

The symptoms of lactose intolerance include abdominal discomfort, bloating and diarrhoea in response to drinking even small amounts of milk. For people with lactose intolerance who wish to drink milk, the enzyme lactase is obtainable from some health food shops as a supplement.

LAUREL, BAY TREE *(Laurus Nobilis)*

An evergreen tree which grows wild in European and Mediterranean countries, the laurel is cultivated for its leathery, lanceolate leaves and fruit. Commonly known as bay leaves, they are commonly used as a flavouring in cooking, but they are astringent and can also be used to stimulate digestion and relieve flatulence. The essential oil (available from larger health food stores in aromatherapy section) made from the fruit and leaves is used for the relief of rheumatism, bruises and skin problems.

LAVENDER *(Lavendula Officinalis)*

A native of the Mediterranean regions, lavender is an evergreen shrub which has for many centuries been widely cultivated for its aromatic flowers. An infusion or the essential oil of the scented flowers is a sedative, and can be used to alleviate cramps and muscle pain. It is also used to treat flatulence, headaches and dizziness. Lavender oil is widely used in aromatherapy and perfumery. Available at larger health food stores in aromatherapy section.

LDL (LOW DENSITY LIPOPROTEINS)

These are a dangerous form of cholesterol carrier which transport **cholesterol** in the bloodstream to the tissues, thus promoting cholesterol deposits, clogging of the arteries, atherosclerosis and heart disease. Lowering LDL levels in the blood can significantly reduce the risk of heart attacks.

LEAD

Lead is a highly toxic element, which even in very small amounts of less than 1 mg a day can be harmful, while larger amounts can be fatal. Its sources in our environment are many and varied: car fumes, industrial emissions and cigarette smoking are just a few. Inhaled lead is most dangerous because it is absorbed in the body much more efficiently than ingested lead.

Lead attacks the brain causing nervousness, depression, apathy, mental retardation in adults and hyperactivity in children. Higher levels of lead poisoning can cause sterility, hypertension and death. Those most at risk are garage workers, painters, plasterers, and workers in battery plants. There are various nutrients which can help to prevent the build-up of lead in the body. For example, **calcium** prevents lead accumulation, **vitamin C** neutralizes lead, **vitamin A** activates the enzymes which prevent lead absorption and **kelp** contains sodium alginate which combines with lead and excretes it through the bowels. Some cases of lead poisoning have been found to respond to penicillamine, a chelating agent which binds with lead, increasing its elimination in the urine.

LECITHIN

Lecithin is a waxy substance found in all body cells and in various foods. It is composed mainly of two B vitamins, phosphatidyl choline and phosphatidyl inositol, and the amino acid methionine. Lecithin is vitally essential to the body: 30 per cent of the brain's dry weight, and 73 per cent of the liver's fat are composed of lecithin.

As a fatty product, lecithin aids transportation of fat throughout the body and, with **cholesterol**, produces bile. Lecithin has a remarkable emulsifying ability. It can help to dissolve minor gallstones, reduce the size of the fatty particles in blood, lower cholesterol levels and prevent atherosclerosis.

Lecithin has been reputed to be a 'brain food' as its ingredient choline is converted in the brain to a neurotransmitter, improving mental function and memory (see CHOLINE). Lecithin supplements can be useful to people engaged in mental work. The best natural sources of lecithin are unrefined, fresh vegetable oils, egg yolks, nuts, seeds and soybeans. Supplemental lecithin made from soybeans is available in granule and capsule forms from health food shops.

LEEK

A vegetable related to the onion, it probably originated in the eastern Mediterranean region. Nowadays, it is popular in northern European countries, especially as a flavouring vegetable in soups and casseroles. It has mild astringent qualities which makes it helpful in the treatment of diarrhoea and internal bleeding.

LEGUMES *(BEANS)*

The Bean family are a group of highly nutritious foods that are an excellent source of complex carbohydrates and dietary fibre. In addition, they provide energy and encourage elimination, and are an inexpensive source of protein, B vitamins and minerals such as calcium, potassium and iron. From a culinary point of view, they are very adaptable and can be prepared in a variety of ways to satisfy most tastes. Sprouted beans (see SPROUTS), which are more easily digested, provide a rich source of vitamin C and enzymes.

When combined with grains in the right proportions, legumes can provide a complete protein that is equal to meat in nutritional value. Members of this food group include black beans, lima beans, kidney beans and pinto beans, adzuki beans, mung beans, peas, chickpeas, lentils, peanuts and soybeans.

LEMON

An excellent source of vitamin C and bioflavonoids, lemon also contains small amounts of calcium, phosphorus, potassium and carotene and, being acidic, can substitute for vinegar in the kitchen. Lemon juice is antiseptic and is a home remedy for many disorders, particularly colds, sore throats, laryngitis, rheumatism, allergies and diarrhoea. It destroys hostile germs, cleanses the blood, promotes weight loss, strengthens weak blood vessels and aids digestion when taken before meals.

Lemon juice is normally used by blending the juice of two average sized lemons with water, to which honey can be added to make it less sharp.

A course of lemon juice treatment can dissolve kidney

stones and gravel when taken on an empty stomach. In this case, the juice of between five to ten lemons should be dissolved in water, which is then sipped throughout the day for a period of two to four weeks.

Fresh lemon can also be used in salad dressings, as lemonade, or as lemon tea, which is made by adding a little lemon juice to a glass of hot water. Lemon rind, too, is very useful: it can be used for flavouring or, if sweetened, it can be eaten on its own as a candy, or with the full lemon. To reap the full benefit of the fruit, it is important to use only fresh lemons, not bottled juice, and to consume them as soon as possible before they spoil.

LEMON BALM *(MELISSA OFFICINALIS)* SEE BALM

LEMON GRASS *(CYMBOPOGON CITRATUS)*

A fragrant tropical grass, it is rich in two volatile (essential) oils, citral and citronellal, and some terpenes. It is used mainly for its antiseptic and antibacterial qualities, but it can also be helpful in the treatment of fever. Scientific studies of lemon grass have found the herb to be an effective treatment for flu and cholera. Available from supermarkets and specialist ethnic grocers.

LENTILS

Lentils are a mildly flavoured legume which come in a great variety of colours and are widely available. India alone produces more than fifty varieties. Generally, however, the green, brown and red varieties are the most commonly used in Western countries. All the varieties are a nutritious source of the B vitamins, iron and fibre. Lentils are the quickest cooking of the legumes. They are also used as sprouts.

LETTUCE

One of the most popular of the salad vegetables, lettuce is rich in vitamins A and C, chlorophyll, iron, potassium and silicone. The darker-leafed varieties contain about six times as much vitamin A and have three times the vitamin C content of the paler varieties such as Iceberg. They are also a better source of potassium.

Lettuce can be used to increase the production of mother's milk, improve urination and help in the treatment of haemorrhoids. Lettuce leaves contain a bitter principle (lactucarium) which is an excellent sedative. A large dish of fresh lettuce leaves eaten before bedtime can calm nervousness and induce sleep.

LEUCINE

Leucine is one of the essential amino acids fundamental to the utilization of protein in the body. It is also one of the three branched chain amino acids and, as such, is used by the body to build and repair muscle tissue. It is also recommended for convalescence after a period of being bedridden. Since leucine lowers blood sugar levels, it must be taken in moderation as it can adversely affect hypoglycaemia.

LICORICE *(Glycyrrhiza Glabra)*

A perennial herb native to southern Europe and Asia, it is also cultivated elsewhere for its root which contains a glycoside (glycyrrhizin) that acts like a mild cortisone. As it is fifty times sweeter than sugar, it is often used to sweeten medicines and also as a flavouring agent. Traditionally, Middle Eastern Arabs used it to prepare a strong infusion called 'soos', which was served cool and used to help digestive disorders.

Licorice tea, or as an infusion, is diuretic and mildly laxative. It is also an expectorant and is used to relieve phlegm. As such, it is commonly used for colds, coughs and mucous congestions. Licorice is also a soothing, emollient herb which can be helpful in healing peptic ulcers. In addition, licorice root, which contains oestrogen precursors, is used in Asian countries for female problems such as irregular menstruation. Licorice is available in health food shops in powder and capsule form, and also as syrups and candies.

LIGNINS

Lignins are types of fibre, found mainly in plant foods such as whole grains, beans, peas, carrots, tomatoes and potatoes. They have various beneficial effects, such as anti-cancer, antibacterial, antiviral and antifungal activity. They can also help to lower high cholesterol levels and prevent the formation of gallstones by binding with the bile acids. Plant lignins are converted in the intestines into two compounds, enterolactone and enterodiol, which protect from cancer. They are especially beneficial in preventing cancer of the colon and breast cancer.

LILY OF THE VALLEY (*Convallaria Majalis*)

A perennial plant, which is found growing wild in Europe and North America in damp, shady places, lily of the valley is also a popular garden plant. It is antispasmodic and diuretic, but is mainly recommended as a heart tonic that can safely strengthen the heart. In larger doses, it can act as a laxative. Available at health food stores and herbalists.

Caution: Lily of the valley should only be used under medical supervision. It contains glycosides which, if taken in incorrect doses, can cause irregular heartbeat and upset stomach.

LINDEN (*Tilia Europaea*)

Also known as lime, this tall, deciduous tree is native to many parts of the northern hemisphere, particularly Europe and North America. An infusion of the leaves and bark is pleasantly aromatic and can be used as a mild sedative. Linden infusions also promote perspiration and are a traditional home remedy for colds, coughs and sore throats. They can also be used as a gargle. Linden flowers produced as a tea provide a delicious and relaxing remedy for stress conditions and is especially good as a bedtime drink. Available at health food stores.

LINSEED OIL SEE FLAX

LIPIDS

A general descriptive term for any group of **fats** or fat-like substances found in the body. This term includes free fatty acids, triglycerides, cholesterol, bile acids, phospholipids and lipoids.

Unless protected by antioxidant nutrients and enzymes, lipids are easily oxidized in the body creating dangerous superoxides and free radicals that attack cells and DNA, and cause heart disease, cancer and other degenerative diseases of ageing.

LIPOIC ACID

A once obscure nutrient, lipoic acid is now rapidly gaining popularity for its many beneficial effects in the body. Lipoic acid, which has many vitamin-like functions, is synthesized in the body, although not always in sufficient quantity. It is a potent antioxidant and a sulphur-containing coenzyme; as such, it is an energizer and plays a vital role in 'burning' blood sugar to energy. It is of benefit to diabetics as it helps to normalize blood sugar levels.

Because lipoic acid is both water-soluble and fat-soluble, it is a universal antioxidant and can also enhance the action of other antioxidant vitamins, such as water-soluble vitamin C and fat-soluble vitamin E. By quenching free radicals, lipoic acid protects cells and helps to prevent the various degenerative diseases of ageing such as heart disease, cancer, diabetes, arthritis, cataracts, Alzheimer's disease, along with many others. It is also a chelating agent – that is, it binds to toxic metals such as lead, cadmium and mercury and removes them from the body.

Lipoic acid supplementation can increase energy and

slow down the ageing process; supplementation is particularly important in later years, when the synthesis of lipoic acid in the body is reduced. Supplementation can also benefit diabetics. Liver and yeast are rich sources of lipoic acid and supplements are available in capsule form from health food stores. The normal daily dose for adults is 20 to 50 mg.

L-METHIONINE SEE METHIONINE

LYSINE

An essential amino acid which is needed to form protein in the body, lysine can effectively suppress the herpes simplex virus (mouth blisters, cold sores) and, because of this, lysine supplements are widely recommended for the treatment of herpes. Lysine is also needed to form collagen, for the subskin and connective tissue, and is essential for calcium absorption.

Since it is lacking in grains, nuts and seeds, lysine supplements (available from health food stores) can help to prevent calcium deficiencies, particularly among strict vegetarians and the elderly. Lysine also combines with methionine, to form carnitine, an important amino acid which aids weight reduction and helps to prevent heart disease.

M

MACADAMIA NUTS

An evergreen tree which is native to tropical Australia, it was taken to Hawaii in the nineteenth century and the nuts are now an important crop there. They are considered by many to be the finest tasting nuts and, since they provide a very concentrated food, rich in natural oils, particularly monounsaturates, they are often used as a substitute for meat. Widely available in supermarkets.

MAGNESIUM

Magnesium is an important mineral which, together with calcium and phosphorus, is found mainly in the bones. Smaller amounts in the blood activate hundreds of enzymes and participate in various biochemical activities. Magnesium maintains strong bones and tooth enamel, calms the nervous system, regulates heartbeat, strengthens digestion, maintains a healthy prostate in men – preventing swelling, keeps calcium soluble – preventing kidney stones, and regulates thyroid function. It also improves urine retention and so helps to control incontinence in the elderly and prevent bed-wetting in children. Magnesium can be depleted in the body by alcohol, sweet foods, and the excessive consumption of milk enriched with vitamin D.

Magnesium deficiencies are manifested in irregular heartbeat and heart attacks, jumpy nerves and weak muscles, convulsions and seizures, prostate enlargement, fatigue, bed-wetting and kidney stones. Its best natural sources include green vegetables, figs, lemons, yellow corn, apples and raw wheat germ. **Dolomite** is a natural supplement.

The normal daily requirement is 350 mg for adults and 250 mg for children; pregnant and lactating women need 450 mg per day. As a supplement, magnesium is available in tablet and capsule form.

MA HUANG (EPHEDRA SINICA)

Ma huang is the Chinese name for ephedra, a low-growing evergreen shrub which is native to the arid and desert regions of the Americas and Asia. It contains ephedrin, an alkaloid which has been shown to reduce excess weight in overweight animals by speeding up the 'burning' of fat into energy and by satisfying hunger. Its action is improved when used with caffeine and theophylline.

Caution: Ma huang has been incorporated as an ingredient in a number of weight loss formulas over the past few years. However, its action is similar to that of adrenalin in that it stimulates the central nervous system, thereby increasing heartbeat and blood pressure. Therefore, ma huang should not be used by hypertensive people or by those with a heart condition.

MAITAKE (GRIFOLA FRONDOSA)

A newly 'rediscovered' ancient mushroom, native to north-east Japan, maitake was traditionally highly prized in Japan both as a culinary and herbal medicine. Oriental folk medicines used it as an important aid to well-being, to maintain health, preserve youth and increase longevity.

The maitake grows in clusters at the base of trees, and in bygone times it was exchanged for its weight in silver. Maitake contains many important vitamins and minerals like B1, B2, B3, C and D, calcium, magnesium, potassium and protein. New research also shows that besides those nutrients, maitake contains a special class of polysaccharides such as beta glucan, and more specifically, its D-fraction. These are complex sugar polymers in maitake extracts, which were found to boost the immune system. Most studies by Japanese scientists, done with the D-fraction of maitake extract, showed maitake to have anti-tumour and anti-cancer activities. Further research is presently being conducted at the Cancer Treatment Center of America to evaluate the anti-cancer properties of maitake.

A recent study in New York with a group of hypertensive human volunteers showed that two 500 mg capsules of maitake a day taken orally for six weeks lowered blood pressure. Dr. Abram Ber, a homeopathic physician from Phoenix, Arizona, is reported to treat hypertension with higher doses: 3 grams maitake per day for the first week, 4 grams per day for the second week, then 5 grams per day as blood pressure indicated, since blood pressure is dose-related.

Other studies have demonstrated maitake's ability to inhibit uterine fibroids, counteract diabetes and even to help lose weight without a change in the diet!

Maitake capsules and tablets, as well as the D-Fractions, are now increasingly being sold in health food stores, as herbal extracts. Maitake is conveniently taken orally. A significant body of research shows that maitake is the most effective of the other medicinal mushrooms such as shiitake and reishi. Maitake doses should best be determined by a qualified practitioner.

MANGANESE

Manganese is a trace element with a wide range of effects. It forms part of many enzymes, such as those involved in sugar metabolism, and is needed to form thyroxine, the thyroid hormone. It also helps in the synthesis of cholesterol and fats, and is important for the production of breast milk and sex hormones, promoting fertility and male potency. Manganese can be used in the prevention of diabetes and nerve-muscle disorders and its best natural sources include whole grains, nuts, green leafy vegetables and tea. The estimated daily requirement is between 2.5 to 5 mg, although lactating women may need up to 9 mg a day. In tea-drinking countries, an average one-third of the daily manganese requirement is obtained from this beverage. Supplements available from health food stores and as multi-vitamin formulas.

MARGARINE

Margarine is made from vegetable oil which undergoes 'hydrogenation'. During this process, hydrogen is added to the oil, saturating its fatty acids and rendering it solid or semi-solid. Saturated fatty acids are not biologically as active as unsaturated ones and they adversely affect cell membranes, leading to various disorders, including high cholesterol levels and diabetes.

The hydrogenation process also changes the structure of the fatty acids from the natural type of cis-fatty acids to the unnatural type of trans-fatty acids which interfere with the utilization of essential fatty acids and, in fact, are not 'recognized' by the body chemistry. For example, they prevent fatty acid transformation to immune cells, inhibiting the synthesis of GLA and prostaglandins (see EVENING

PRIMROSE OIL). In the US and the UK, most of the consumption of trans-fatty acid consists of margarine and shortening.

MARJORAM (*MAJORANA HORTENSIS*)

A scented herb, it is both an annual and a perennial, and was originally native to northern African and south-western Asia. Nowadays, it is widely cultivated as a popular culinary herb and is available from supermarkets and grocers. Sweet marjoram tea is pleasantly carminative. It can relieve flatulence and colic in children – upset stomach and gastritis can be soothed, both internally and externally, by massaging the abdomen with a clockwise rotation. The essential oil of sweet marjoram is also used externally for arthritis, gout, rheumatism and varicose veins. It is claimed to have a calming effect and can be used to alleviate grief.

Caution: Marjoram should not be used during pregnancy.

MARSHMALLOW (*ALTHEA OFFICINALIS*)

A wild, perennial plant with soft hairy leaves, it is found mainly in marshy areas and damp, watery places. Marshmallow leaves and roots have long been known for their demulcent, soothing and softening properties and infusions prepared from the plant are excellent for the treatment of coughs, cystitis and for soothing the digestive tract in cases of ulcers. Externally, a poultice prepared from the leaves steeped in boiling water can be applied to boils and abscesses.

MATÉ *(ILEX PARAGUAYENSIS)*

Also called Paraguay tea, maté tea is a stimulating beverage made from the dried leaves of a South American oak which is very popular in Latin America. The dried leaves are also exported and are available in many health food stores. Maté tea has a high caffeine content and is renowned as a tonic and stimulant, increasing alertness and mental acuity. It contains iron and is useful in the treatment of iron-deficiency anaemia. It is also a diuretic, stimulating the kidneys, and alleviating arthritis and gout. Maté tea is very satisfying and can help slimmers to lose excess weight. Once made, the tea should be drunk fresh as it becomes black and bitter if allowed to stand.

Caution: People with cardiovascular or nervous conditions, or those allergic to caffeine, should avoid maté. Excessive consumption can cause diarrhoea.

MEDIUM CHAIN TRIGLYCERIDES (MCTs)

MCTs are a special type of saturated fat derived from coconut oil which are used by the body differently to most other fats. In the main, fats such as butter, margarine, animal fats and even edible oils are composed of long chain triglycerides (LCTs), which are absorbed into the lymph system and stored for future use. They take a long time to be converted into energy. MCTs, on the other hand, have much shorter molecules so that they can pass easily through the liver and are directly absorbed into the bloodstream. In this way, they are converted much more rapidly into utilized energy rather than being deposited as fat.

MCTs have been found to promote weight loss, increase energy and are also useful for treating epilepsy. They are now increasingly available in supplements and also as MCT oils, which can be used in the kitchen in the same way as any of the other edible oils.

MEADOW SAFFRON *(Colchicum Autumnale)*

A perennial herb which grows wild in damp places, but is also cultivated in the US for its bulb and seeds. It contains colchicine, a poisonous alkaloid, which inhibits cell multiplication. It is used medicinally in very tiny amounts in the treatment of gout and arthritis.

Caution: The whole herb is poisonous and must not be used as a home remedy.

MEAT

Meat is the principal provider of high-quality protein and fat with other important vitamins such as B12 and minerals such as zinc. Organ meats, like liver, heart and kidneys, are the most nutritious. Generally, meat is considered a tonic: blood-building and helping relieve general weakness. However, its metabolic by-products in the body are very toxic. People on meat-centered-diets are often thirsty; they need fluids to flush these toxins out. More and more studies published in the media are advising the public to cut down on red meat.

With higher standards of living in the West meat consumption soared. The accelerating incidence of heart disease and cancer has been linked with increased beef consumption, which has increased from 60 pounds per person in 1950 to almost 150 pounds today. Beef in the fifties provided more nutrients and was much leaner, with 5 to 10 per cent carcass fat, largely unsaturated. Today's cattle, intensively raised on high-energy feeds, deprived of grazing and treated with antibiotic drugs, hormones and tranquilisers, have 30 per cent fat. Most of these drugs, hormones and pesticide sprays accumulate in this fat. Meat is often treated with nitrites and nitrates which are used to preserve it. These can combine in the stomach to form nitrosamines, potent carcinogens that were found to produce cancer in rats after only one dose. Processed ground meat products like sausages and hot dogs are the most dangerous, since poor grade meats and preservatives which can be used in their preparation are hard to detect in these highly seasoned products.

Livers of beef, calf, veal, lamb and pork have been known to strengthen the body in stressful conditions. Chicken liver is known to strengthen both liver and kidneys; helpful in treating conditions such as iron-deficiency anaemia, impotence, tendency to miscarry, blurred vision and urinary incontinence. Desiccated liver tablets are available at health food stores.

MELATONIN

Melatonin is a natural hormone secreted mainly in the pineal gland, a pea-size gland in the mid-brain. It is in fact produced by pineal enzymes that are respectively activated and depressed by darkness and light. As a result, the pineal increases its secretion of melatonin during darkness, thus inducing sleep. As a natural sleeping aid, melatonin swept the world during the early 1990s, and melatonin supplements (sold in health food stores and pharmacies) in potencies of 1 to 3 mg are now widely used in the US to combat jet lag and insomnia. Melatonin is also thought to alleviate depression while, in addition, it has also been found to be a powerful antioxidant. As such, it boosts the immune system and stimulates the production of antibodies and other immune cells that fight disease, especially the degenerative diseases of ageing such as heart disease and cancer. Melatonin is widely used in the USA as a supplement in health food stores. In the UK it is discontinued in health food stores but is still available as a prescription drug. (It is still a controversial supplement).

MELISSA see BALM

MERCURY

Mercury is a toxic element and a common pollutant. Its main sources are fish, pesticides, fungistats (which prevent mould in seeds) and emissions from coal burning. The mercury which pollutes lakes and oceans is methyl mercury, a compound which is fifty times more toxic than pure mercury. Methyl mercury is dumped into rivers and lakes by various industrial plants, such as paper mills which use mercury to protect paper from mould. As a result of this dumping, fish can become a highly concentrated source of mercury. For example, in Lake Erie irreversible pollution with mercury has occurred in such high levels that fishing has been strictly prohibited.

A build-up of mercury in the body can cause damage to the brain, kidneys and nervous system resulting in, for example, paralysis and blindness. The commonest sources of mercury in everyday life are batteries, mercury vapour lamps, dental fillings and mercury thermometers. Some nutrients, such as selenium, counteract mercury in the body. Among the other protective nutrients are calcium, vitamins A, C, E and B complex, lecithin and stomach acid, which is sold as betaine HCl capsules.

METHIONINE, L-METHIONINE

Methionine is an essential amino acid needed for the synthesis of protein in the body. It is a sulphur-containing amino acid and a lipotropic, which means that it has an affinity to fats. As such, it helps to produce **lecithin**, which emulsifies fats and breaks down fatty deposits, preventing their build-up in the liver and arteries and thus reducing the risk of heart and circulatory diseases.

Methionine is a strong detoxifier and combines with toxic elements such as lead, cadmium and mercury to eliminate them from the body, preventing many related conditions such as hypertension, depression and kidney damage. It is also a strong antioxidant, neutralizing the free radicals which oxidize cells and which are the underlying cause for the degenerative diseases of ageing, such as heart disease, cancer and diabetes. Methionine also strengthens muscles and helps to prevent hair loss. It is available as a food supplement in health food shops.

MILK

Milk was once promoted as the 'perfect food' and, indeed, cow's milk is an excellent source of protein and the best nutritional source of calcium. It also provides fat which aids the absorption of calcium and its phosphorus content offers an ideal calcium–phosphorus ratio which is required for calcium utilization. In addition, milk contains a good balance of vitamins A, D, E, K and B2, and a litre (2 pints) of milk a day can supply approximately all the required calcium, phosphorus and fat. Milk is a fully digestible food except for those people who are unable to digest milk sugar (**lactose intolerance**).

However, milk has its drawbacks. It is low in vitamin C, iron and copper, and is increasingly considered to be a polluted food in that it may contain residues of pesticides, hormones, DDT, steroids and antibiotics (used in udder inflammations). It is also a common allergen and there are many people, including children, who must avoid it. Nevertheless, for most people, milk remains a nourishing food, although many nutritionists now advise that the average daily intake should be less than previously recommended.

However, cow's milk cannot be considered a good substitute for human milk. Compared to mother's milk, cow's milk is deficient in vitamins A, B1, C and E; its mineral content is three times that of mother's milk and contained in different proportions, and it has more protein and bigger fat globules, which are suited to raising calves, but not human babies. The type of lactose in cow's milk (alpha lactose) does not encourage the growth of intestinal flora in babies as does the lactose contained in mother's milk (beta lactose).

Goat's milk is a much more tolerable and suitable form of milk for babies than that of cows. In fact, since the time of Hippocrates, physicians have recommended goat's milk for infants and convalescents because it is so easily digested. Compared to cow's milk, goat's milk has less protein, smaller fat globules, a little more calcium and vitamin A, and nearly ten times the fluorine needed to build strong bones and teeth. Goat's milk is usually given to infants who are allergic to cow's milk or who cannot tolerate the mother's milk. Although goat's milk provides less than 3 per cent of the world milk supply, whole populations in Asia and Africa consume it because 70 per cent of the world's goats are found in those countries.

MILK THISTLE (*CARDUUS MARIANUS*)

An annual plant which grows wild in dry, rocky soils in parts of Europe and North America, its leaves provide a bitter tonic and its seeds contain flavones (silydanin and silymarin) which stimulate the evacuation of bile. Both the leaves and seeds can also be used in the treatment of liver diseases and to protect the liver from toxins. Milk thistle can be very beneficial in the treatment of hepatitis and cirrhosis of the liver. It is now available in capsules from herbalists and is also found in major health food shops.

MINT SEE PEPPERMINT

MISO

A savoury fermented *soybean* paste, used for seasoning, miso has traditionally been used in China and Japan for many thousands of years. Miso soup is a popular dish in Japanese and Chinese restaurants. Miso is made from cooked soybeans, grain (barley or rice), salt and water which are combined with a mould starter. The mixture is then allowed to ferment for between six months and a year.

Miso comes in many varieties and colours and, because it is usually very salty, can be used as a substitute for salt or soy sauce. As a result of fermentation, it is a live food, containing friendly micro-organisms which are beneficial to the intestinal flora. It is therefore best consumed uncooked. Many varieties of miso are available in health food shops.

MISTLETOE *(VISCUM ALBUM)*

An evergreen, semi-parasitic plant which grows on the branches of host trees, it has long been revered as a sacred plant in many European religions and closely associated with magic and healing. Both the leaves and berries are known to be useful in the regulation of blood pressure, both for high and low high blood pressure. Mistletoe has also been used as a nerve tonic in the treatment of tension, insomnia and depression and, prepared as a tea from the leaves and berries, it is a diuretic and stimulant and can be used for strengthening the heart.

Caution: Mistletoe is potentially toxic and should not be used in doses greater than 4 g of the crude herb, or for extended periods, except under the supervision of a naturopath. Available at health food stores and herbalists and as formulas.

MOLASSES

Molasses is a concentrated syrup, a by-product of sugar refining, which precipitates as residue after the sugar crystals have been separated from the sugar-cane juice. Molasses is rich in nutrients and low in sugar and, in fact, the nutrients in molasses are 30 times more concentrated than in the original cane juice. It provides an excellent source of minerals and trace elements, including iron, calcium, potassium, magnesium, copper, chromium, manganese, molybdenum and zinc. One tablespoonful of molasses supplies as much calcium as a glass of milk and as much iron as nine eggs. Molasses also contains high levels of B vitamins, and is an alkali-forming food. It is reported to have a beneficial effect on many conditions such as anaemia, fatigue, arthritis, ulcers and colitis. It also has a strong laxative effect and is used to counteract constipation. Unsulphured molasses is better than that preserved with sulphur, and crude black molasses is preferable to the sweeter varieties. A normal intake is one to three teaspoonfuls a day.

Note: It is recommended that teeth are rinsed after taking molasses because, like sugar, molasses can cause tooth decay.

Available at health food stores.

MOLYBDENUM

Molybdenum is a trace element widely present in raw foods and an essential part of several important enzymes. Molybdenum prevents tooth decay and anaemia, and is also thought to prevent oesophageal cancer and increase sexual potency in older men. Since most of the molybdenum content is lost during the milling of whole grains and the refining of raw sugar, a diet based on these refined foods can result in a deficiency. The best natural sources of molybdenum are legumes, whole grain cereals and dark green leafy vegetables, and a balanced diet should supply adequate amounts of it.

MONOSODIUM GLUTAMATE (*MSG*)

As a food ingredient, MSG is a flavour enhancer which deserves a special mention since it is commonly used in many processed foods (E621), and especially in Chinese restaurants. An amino acid, MSG is the sodium salt of glutamic acid (620).

MSG was first isolated at the Tokyo University in 1908, from a seaweed (Laminaria Japonica) which was long known by Japanese cooks to improve food taste. Initially considered safe, MSG was linked to many allergic symptoms often referred to as 'Chinese Restaurant Syndrome' because they were observed mainly after eating Chinese. These symptoms include thirst and nausea, water retention, muscle numbness, palpitation, dizziness, headaches or a cold sweat.

It is estimated that some 25 per cent of the Western population are allergic to MSG, in one way or the other. Anyone allergic to MSG should realise that while some food labels may claim No MSG, the presence of MSG can be disguised with vague or technical language, such as: glutamic acid; natural flavours; seasoning; modified food starch; autolyzed food yeast.

MUSHROOMS

Fungi which, in the wild, grow most commonly in woods and damp grassy areas, the cultivated varieties are available all the year round. Mushrooms of the button variety are rich in potassium, phosphorus, copper and iron. They are also a good source of thiamine (vitamin B1) and riboflavin (vitamin B2). As mushrooms mature, their caps open and expose their gills. It is best to avoid wide open caps and also to select mushrooms that are firm, not spongy.

Mushrooms are known to be beneficial in reducing blood fat levels and to have antibiotic properties; they are also claimed to have anti-tumour activity and to boost the immune system action against disease-producing micro-organisms by increasing white blood cell count. Mushrooms are easily digested and are recommended for anyone suffering with digestive problems.

MUSTARD *(BRASSICA NIGRA)*

An annual plant that is native to the temperate regions of the northern hemisphere, it is also widely cultivated for its seeds which contain a strong volatile oil. Mustard is a popular culinary herb that stimulates the appetite and helps digestion. A weak tea of mustard seeds can be used, in small amounts, for bronchitis or coughs. For external applications, mustard is used mainly as an irritant to promote blood flow in cases of rheumatism and colds. Mustard seed powder is mixed with wheat flour and water to form a thick paste and this is then spread on a linen cloth to form a poultice, which is laid on the affected area causing the skin to heat up. The poultice must not be used on sensitive areas and it should be removed when the heat becomes too uncomfortable. Wheat flour is added in order to reduce the warming effects of the mustard, and its quantity in the poultice should be adjusted according to the amount of warming desired. Diluted mustard seed oil can also be used externally for similar conditions.

N

NAC *(N-ACETYL CYSTEINE)*

N-acetyl cysteine is a powerful antioxidant which provides protection from free radical damage. It strengthens resistance to diseases by increasing immune cells in blood. It combats viruses and was studied for its ability to inhibit the AIDS virus. It is normally prescribed for bronchitis and, as a sulphur-containing compound, NAC detoxifies the liver and helps its function. Available at health food stores.

NETTLE, STINGING *(URTICA DIOICA)*

Although a coarse herb which grows freely as a weed across Europe, Asia and North America, the leaves, flowers and seeds of the stinging nettle contain a wide range of useful medicinal and culinary properties. The plant makes an effective tonic and can be used to promote appetite and eliminate intestinal worms, while its fresh juice will stimulate digestion and promote milk flow in nursing mothers. It is also an astringent and can inhibit urinary tract bleeding, haemorrhoids and excessive menstrual flow. As a decoction, nettle can be used to strengthen the hair and, when used as a wash, to rejuvenate the skin. The leaves of the nettle, which are rich in vitamins and minerals, are often used to flavour salads and make infusions.

Caution: As its name implies, the plant should be handled with care. The fresh leaves are covered with bristly hairs which, when touched, will inject an irritant substance into the skin. However, the irritant loses its effect a few hours after picking, and is destroyed with cooking.

NEUROTRANSMITTERS (*NT*)

Neurotransmitters are special chemicals which carry messages between brain cells. All learning, remembering, sleeping and emotions depend upon the ability of the brain cells to produce and deliver neurotransmitters to other brain cells, as well as to respond to messages from other brain cells.

Neurotransmitters are produced from nutrients absorbed from food. For example, acetylcholine, which is needed by the brain for learning, memory and long-term planning, is made in the body from choline, a B vitamin found in egg yolks, grains, legumes, green leafy vegetables, and from lecithin which is rich in phosphatidyl choline. Another neurotransmitter, norepinephrine (brain adrenalin), which is needed for wakefulness, sex, learning and body movement, is produced in the brain by phenylalanine and tyrosine, two amino acids that are found in meat, eggs and cheese. A deficiency of norepinephrine can cause stress, depression and low sex drive. Other important neurotransmitters include dopamine, **GABA**, **melatonin** and **serotonin**. Some neurotransmitters, such as norepinephrine, have an excitatory action, while others such as serotonin, have a calming effect.

NIACIN SEE VITAMIN B3

NIGHTSHADES

The nightshades are a class of vegetables including potatoes, tomatoes, aubergine, peppers and tobacco. They all contain solanin, a toxic alkaloid which can cause headaches, osteoarthritis, diarrhoea, and vomiting in sensitive people. Solanine is usually neutralized by cooking, baking, roasting or frying.

NITRATES, NITRITES

These are chemicals which are used to treat and preserve bacon and other meats, to give them an attractive red colouring and to prevent botulism and aflatoxin mould. Nitrates are toxic as they react with protein to form nitrosamines, which are cancer-causing substances. However, this risk can be reduced by taking supplemental vitamin C.

NORI

A seaweed with fibrous, jade-coloured fronds, nori has the highest protein content of all the seaweeds (48 per cent dry weight) and is also rich in iodine, sodium, vitamins A, B1 and niacin. It can help in the treatment of goitre, and is also used to reduce cholesterol levels, alleviate painful urination, reduce high blood pressure and aid digestion. It is sold in sheets in health food stores and used in cooking.

NUCLEIC ACIDS

Nucleic acids are special proteins which contain the genetic code and heredity information for the human body. They are present in all cells and supervise their growth, multiplication and functioning. They consist of DNA (deoxyribonucleic acid), which contains the master 'blueprint', and RNA (ribonucleic acid), which acts as the messenger to the cells. Nucleic acids are vulnerable to free radical damage in that free radicals oxidize the nucleic acids and cross-link their molecules, distorting their information. This distorted information can lead to mutations in cell multiplication and performance, cancer and premature ageing. DNA and RNA can be protected by **antioxidant** vitamins and nutrients. Nucleic acids are available as nutritional supplements.

Caution: Nucleic acid supplements are not suitable for people with gout as they increase uric acid levels.

NUTMEG *(MYRISTICA FRAGRANS)*

A tropical evergreen tree that is native to the Molucca (Spice) Islands, it is now cultivated in Indonesia, the West Indies, Brazil, India and Sri Lanka for its aromatic seeds which are used mainly as a culinary spice, also known as mace. The ground seeds improve appetite, stimulate digestion and relieve flatulence. It is also a mild hallucinogenic.

Caution: Eating nutmeg in more than seasoning amounts can be dangerous. Overdoses can produce poisoning symptoms such as stomach pain, dizziness and delirium. Widely available ground or whole in supermarkets.

OATS *(Avena Sativa)*

Oats are an exceptional cereal and are used primarily for their outstanding nutritional value. They are a few times higher in protein and fat content than any other cereal and are also rich in vitamin E, some of the B vitamins and minerals, particularly zinc, manganese and silica. They are high in fibre and, prepared as a porridge, can help to prevent constipation, soothe the digestive system, remove cholesterol and strengthen the heart. They are also useful in conditions such as weakness, diabetes, hepatitis, indigestion and bloating. Oats help to strengthen bones as they are rich in silica, and a tincture of oats has been reported to reduce cravings for cigarettes. In addition to porridge, oats are also used in soups, puddings, breads and desserts.

OCTACOSANOL

An ingredient of wheat germ oil, it has been found to increase energy, endurance and strength by increasing oxygen utilization in muscles during exercise. Octacosanol also benefits muscular dystrophy and other nerve–muscle disorders. It is now available on its own or incorporated into nutritional formulas (see WHEAT GERM OIL).

OLIVE OIL

One of the most desirable oils, especially when it is extra virgin, cold pressed and unrefined, the main fatty acid in olive oil, oleic acid, is monounsaturated, omega-9 fatty acid. It is less vulnerable to rancidity and more resistant to heat than polyunsaturated oils, such as safflower and corn, and is therefore highly recommended for cooking. It is also excellent used fresh as a salad dressing. Olive oil is a popular remedy in Mediterranean countries for gallstones; it also helps to flush out kidney stones, and is used for constipation and to lower high cholesterol levels. Olive oil can be also used externally to treat burns, bruises and sprains.

OLIVE TREE LEAVES

A food and medicine since biblical times, olive leaves have now been 'rediscovered' as an energizing food with antiviral and antibacterial properties. As far back as 1855, information started to spread that drinking bitter tea brewed from olive tree leaves was a potential cure for malaria. More recently, the active ingredients in the leaves, two phenolic compounds (oleuropein and elenolate), have been isolated. Oleuropein has been found to inhibit two types of fermentative bacteria – which, incidentally, is why olives are often cracked before pickling and the phenols removed, since they inhibit fermentation.

Olive leaf extract is increasingly used as a supplement to treat chronic fatigue and boost the immune system. It is also recommended for sore throats, coughs and sinus problems. Oleuropein has been found to be an effective antioxidant, preventing cholesterol from oxidization. As such, it is used to reduce the risk of coronary heart disease in vulnerable people, since oxidized cholesterol is easily deposited, causing blocked blood vessels. Olive leaf extract is now available in capsule form from the Allergy Research Group in San Leandro CA, USA.

OMEGA-3 FATTY ACIDS

These are types of essential, polyunsaturated fatty acids. They include EPA (eicosapentaenoic acid) and DHA (docosahexaenoic acid) which are found mainly in ocean fish like salmon, mackerel and sardines, and ALA (alpha-linolenic acid) found mainly in flaxseed oil. The omega-3 fatty acids are very important to the body's health. They reduce blood stickiness, blood clotting, cholesterol levels, blood pressure and inflammations. In this way they help to prevent heart attacks and strokes.

ALA can be converted in the body to EPA, and similarly, EPA can be converted to DHA. EPA however, is considered the most beneficial of the omegas. It is the best source for the body's own production of beneficial prostaglandins that also help reduce inflammations. As such, EPA is considered very helpful in heart disease and inflammatory conditions like arthritis, and is the reason why heart patients and arthritics are often advised to eat ocean fish instead of meat. EPA is now also available in capsule form, and is sold as a food supplement in health food stores. DHA is particularly important for the eye tissue and for brain development in infancy.

ONION

Probably first grown in central or south-western Asia, nowadays onions are grown throughout the world, mainly for their culinary properties, although for many centuries they have been recognized also for their medicinal value. The healing properties of onions are now scientifically established and are attributed to their many important components, such as **quercetin**, mustard oils and sulphur-containing compounds. Onions can reduce blood stickiness, preventing blood clots and heart attacks. Crude extracts of onion have been shown to lower high blood pressure and cholesterol levels. Onions are also used to expel phlegm and alleviate coughs, colds and inflammations of nose and throat. Onion tea is calming and acts as a general sedative.

ORANGE

The orange is among the oldest cultivated fruits known to man and has been grown for more than 4,000 years. It probably originated in the south-western regions of Asia, but nowadays is cultivated in subtropical climates worldwide.

Orange is an acidic fruit, which is best known for its high vitamin C content – 60 mg per 100 g edible fruit – which is always highest in the early part of the season and much lower in the late season. Oranges also contain vitamin A, potassium, calcium, phosphorus and folic acid. The white part of the rind is a rich source of **pectin** which lowers cholesterol and of **bioflavonoids**, and benefits weak gums, capillaries and blood vessels. In fact, sweetened orange peel is a popular Middle-Eastern treat. The fruit itself has strong anti-inflammatory effects and can be used as a general tonic; it improves digestion and is beneficial for conditions such as colds, arthritis and fevers. The oil derived from the orange rind can relieve flatulence.

OREGANO (ORIGANUM VULGARE)

A perennial herb, native to the Mediterranean regions, oregano is commonly used as a culinary spice. Infusions of the leaves, flowers and stalks can benefit an upset stomach, colic, headaches, nervousness, coughs, whooping cough and other respiratory disorders. Oregano also promotes perspiration, relieves flatulence and expels phlegm. Oregano tea can be used to relieve abdominal cramps in women and regulate the menstrual cycle when taken three or four days before the period is due.

Caution: Oregano should not be used during pregnancy.

ORNITHINE, L-ORNITHINE

Ornithine is derived from **arginine**, and shares its properties in that it is a growth hormone releaser and strengthens the immune system. However, supplemental ornithine should be taken in half the quantities recommended for arginine.

OXALIC ACID

Oxalic acid is a nutrient found in various vegetables and fruits, particularly in spinach, rhubarb, beets and cranberries; it is also found in chocolate. Consumption of oxalic acid-containing foods can increase any tendency to kidney stones or gravel since the oxalic acid in the food may combine with calcium, resulting in calcium–oxalate kidney stones. People with a known tendency to kidney stones or gravel would therefore do well to cut down on the amount of oxalic acid–containing foods in their diet.

OKR A

A native of Africa, okra – also known as gumbo or bamia – is grown in large quantities in the southern states of the US. It is also very popular in Middle–Eastern cooking. An annual, the vegetable is produced for its green pods which contain large amounts of vitamins A and C, calcium, phosphorus, potassium and magnesium. The plant is also rich in mucilaginous substances which lubricate the intestines and are recommended for soothing duodenal ulcers and reducing high cholesterol levels.

OYSTERS

Found mainly in oceans and coastal regions with mild to tropical climates, oysters are one of the richest sources of zinc and are often recommended as an aphrodisiac, to increase fertility and sex drive. Fresh oysters contain 149 mg zinc per 100 g of the edible portions. The shell is a rich source of calcium and is sometimes used in calcium supplements.

Caution: Because of their zinc content, oysters should only be eaten in moderation.

P

PABA *(Para Amino Benzoic Acid)*

An **antioxidant** vitamin which is related to **folic acid**, PABA is the 'sun screen' vitamin which protects the skin from sunburn. It is known for its ability to absorb ultra violet (UV) light, thus preventing wrinkling of the skin and reducing the risk of skin cancer. It is therefore widely used in sunblock preparations.

PABA also has other beneficial effects. It corrects loss of pigmentation in skin and hair, prevents hair greying and retards hair loss. It also protects the lungs from ozone damage, acts as a **coenzyme** in the utilization of **protein** and assists the formation of red blood cells.

Deficiency symptoms include skin conditions such as eczema and wrinkles, fatigue, irritability and depression, senility, arthritis and bursitis. Among its best natural sources are organ meats, brewer's yeast, whole grains, raw wheat germ and molasses. No recommended daily allowances have been established, but an allowance of between 30 mg and 100 mg is considered reasonable. In spite of the fact that the body synthesizes PABA, it may not be sufficient for maximum protection and therefore PABA supplements can usefully enhance its beneficial effects.

PANCREATIN

This is the name of digestive-aid tablets containing pancreatic enzymes such as protease, lipase and amylase. These enzymes breakdown proteins, fats and starch, and assist in their digestion. Pancreatin tablets can prevent bloating, stomach discomfort, indigestion and gastroenteritis (inflammation of stomach and intestines), and are normally taken after main meals to strengthen digestion. Since the secretion of digestive enzymes is reduced with age, pancreatin tablets are often recommended by nutritionists for even healthy people over 40. Pancreatin can also prevent food allergies that arise from by-products of incomplete digestion.

PANGAMIC ACID

Pangamic acid, or vitamin B15, is used mainly in Russia to improve heart conditions and athletic performance. It is still not fully officially accepted in the West. It is an antioxidant and prevents the formation of destructive superoxide radicals, a major cause of ageing. It is also an antipollutant, eliminating environmental toxins from the body. Being a lipotropic substance, it lowers cholesterol levels and prevents fat accumulation in the liver. A deficiency of pangamic acid can cause reduced oxygenation of the blood, leading to fatigue and lowered fitness. Its best natural sources are brewer's yeast, brown rice, whole grains, pumpkin and sesame seeds. There are no recommended daily allowances, but a daily intake of 25 to 100 mg is normal. It is sometimes available as a supplement called 'calcium pangamate'.

PANTOTHENIC ACID

Although pantothenic acid, also called vitamin B5, occurs in small amounts in most foods, a deficiency of the vitamin is commonplace. It is involved in a number of metabolic functions, such as fat and sugar metabolism and the production of adrenalin, which is needed in stress conditions. It also helps to maintain normal blood sugar levels, and increase energy, particularly in stressful situations – which is why it is often called the 'stress vitamin'; it is also used to treat rheumatoid arthritis and allergies. Pantothenic acid is an important ingredient of royal jelly and cod's roe – hence its use for improving fertility and reproduction.

Some indications of a deficiency of the vitamin include stress, irritability or depression, low blood sugar levels, fatigue, indigestion, constipation, ulcers, arthritis and allergies. Among the best natural sources are royal jelly, cod's roe, brewer's yeast, organ meats, raw wheat germ, whole grains, beans, molasses and nuts.

The recommended daily allowance for pantothenic acid is set at 10 mg, but most nutritionists recommend 30 to 50 mg a day. It is available as supplement on its own, and is also included in B complex and multivitamin supplements

PAPAIN SEE PAPAYA

PAPAYA, PAWPAW, PAPAIN (CARICA PAPAYA)

A sweet tropical fruit, which is eaten fresh and is best known for its ability to aid digestion. Papaya contains the enzyme papain which helps to digest proteins and is therefore useful for the relief of dyspepsia and weak digestion. It is also helpful in cases of food allergies caused by incomplete digestion of protein fragments. In tropical regions, papaya has long been used as a meat tenderizer, and it is also known to expel worms, treat dysentery and relieve rheumatic pain. Papaya is a rich source of beta carotene (provitamin A) and vitamins B and C, making it a very nutritious food. It is increasingly used in the manufacture of commercial digestive aids and skin creams.

PARSLEY

Parsley is a very popular biennial herb with aromatic leaves that is used as a culinary flavouring. The leaves are either eaten fresh in salads or steeped for tea. Parsley is an excellent diuretic and is useful for kidney disorders and the elimination of stones and gravel. Both the fresh juice, as well as a tea made from the leaves or seeds, can be used to relieve water retention (oedema) and strengthen digestion. Parsley also stimulates delayed menstruation and promotes menstrual flow.

PARSNIP

A sweet culinary root vegetable which is mildly diuretic, it lubricates the intestines and is beneficial for soothing stomach and intestinal irritations. It helps to clean the liver and gall bladder and, used in soups or teas, it promotes perspiration and is beneficial for coughs, colds, headaches and arthritis.

Caution: Only the root part of the plant should be eaten. Parsnip leaves are poisonous.

PASSION FLOWER *(Passiflora incarnata)*

A strong climbing vine which grows wild and is also cultivated as a garden plant, the flowers are used mainly to calm
nervousness and hysteria, relieve headaches and induce
sleep. A tea (available from health food stores) prepared from
the flowers is effective against involuntary cramps and for
high blood pressure caused by nervous conditions. The fruit
is sold as a delicacy in some shops and can be used for con-
serving and flavouring.

PAU D'ARCO *(Tabevulia)*

A South American bitter herb which is antibacterial, anti-
fungal and a booster of the immune system. It has traditionally been used to control candida (thrush) and help in the
treatment of cancer. It is also used to cleanse the blood, treat
liver disease, infections, diabetes, ulcers, allergies and
tumours. Pau d'arco is available as tea bags in many health
food shops.

PAWPAW SEE PAPAYA

PEAS

Native to temperate climates, fresh peas are sweet and juicy,
and one of the most easily digestible and non-gassy
legumes. They contain 78 per cent water, with only traces
of fat, are low in sodium and provide a good source of iron
and vitamins A, C, B1, B2 and niacin. Peas have a diuretic

and mildly laxative effect and are recommended for strengthening digestion, reducing water retention and helping to promote elimination. They are popular as a summer vegetable and also make a nutritious addition to salads, soups and casseroles.

PEACH

A deciduous tree, grown in temperate climates, it is believed that the peach was originally native to China where it has been grown for several thousand years. It was spread throughout Europe by the Romans and first taken to North America in the sixteenth century by the Spanish explorers. Peaches are a delicious fruit, providing a rich source of beta carotene, iron and calcium, together with some vitamin C and niacin. The fruit is astringent and tends to limit perspiration. It can also be used to alleviate coughs and gastrointestinal inflammations.

PEANUTS

A legume which is now grown throughout the warm regions of the world, particularly in Africa and Asia, the peanut was originally native to South America. Peanuts are high in fat (oil), and rich in protein, niacin, calcium and magnesium. Due to their high oil content, they are best eaten raw or slightly roasted and since they contain almost 49 per cent fat, they are not very suitable for dieters. Peanuts lubricate the intestines and are useful for the alleviation of ulcers or digestive tract tumours. They are known to increase milk flow in nursing mothers, to curb internal bleedings and improve hearing. A tea made from the shells was traditionally used to lower high blood pressure. Eaten in moderation, peanuts can benefit underweight people.

Caution: Large amounts can cause skin problems. Peanuts are a heavily sprayed nut and are subject to aflatoxin, a carcinogenic fungus. It is safer, therefore, to eat organically-grown peanuts.

PEAR

Closely related to the apple and the quince, pears are grown throughout the temperate regions of the world. The fruit is high in water and fibre, but low in vitamin C and minerals and can be used to alleviate constipation, coughs and sore throats; the fibre will soothe intestinal inflammations. However, excessive use of pears is not recommended, especially during pregnancy, since their fibre taxes digestion.

PECAN

Native to North America, the tree is grown throughout the southern states of the US and, to a lesser extent, in South Africa, Australia and the Middle East. It is valued for its fruit, the pecan nut, which is rich in fat, and provides one of the highest sources of unsaturated fatty acids. Seventy-seven per cent of its total calories come from its fat content. The pecan nut is therefore very calorific and although, nutritionally, it is high in potassium and B vitamins, it contains far too many calories for the amount of protein it provides. Pecans are delicious and best eaten fresh before their oils become rancid but, due to their high calorific value, they are not very suitable for anyone who is overweight or on a weight-reducing diet.

PECTIN

Pectin is a gel-forming dietary fibre which forms part of plant cells and is found mainly in the skins, peels and rinds of fruits and vegetables. Orange rind contains 30 per cent pectin, apple peel 15 per cent and onion skin 12 per cent. Pectin has several nutritional roles: binds cholesterol and bile acids in the intestines, promoting their excretion, thus helping lower high cholesterol levels; pectin also binds with toxic metals such as lead, mercury and cadmium, and with radioactive residues, and excretes them from the body. Pectin supplements sold in health food stores have been found to be helpful in controlling diabetes, treating constipation and reducing the risk of heart attacks. Pectin is also used as a stabiliser and thickener (E440b) in commercially processed jams and preserves.

PEPPERS

Originating in South America and brought to Europe in the sixteenth century, the pepper is now grown throughout much of the world – as a perennial in tropical regions and, in temperate areas, as an annual. The colourful fruit of the plant – its red, green and yellow peppers, or capsicums – provide an excellent source of beta carotene and vitamin C; they also contain high amounts of calcium, phosphorus, sodium and potassium. Peppers can improve appetite and digestion, promote circulation and reduce swellings.

Caution: Peppers are a known allergen which can cause reactions in many people. If an allergy is suspected, it is best to avoid peppers for a week, then try them again to check for any recurrence of symptoms. Usually, people allergic to raw peppers will find they can safely eat them if cooked.

PEPPERMINT, MINT

A perennial herb of the mint family, which grows best in moist soils, it is widely cultivated in the temperate regions of Europe and North America. The herb contains menthol and is popular both as a flavouring agent and as a tea. It is also well known for its carminative effects – that is, it helps to relieve flatulence and indigestion. Since menthol is also an appetite stimulant, digestive and sedative, peppermint can be used to prevent or alleviate cramps, insomnia and vomiting; it is also claimed to be an aphrodisiac. In addition, peppermint has antiviral properties: its tannins have been found to suppress the activity of the flu virus and inhibit Herpes simplex. Peppermint oil is used to relieve the symptoms of irritable bowel syndrome (IBS).

PERSIMMON

A small tree that belongs to the ebony family, two of its species are grown for their pulpy, edible fruits. One of these, the kaki or Japanese persimmon, is native to central and northern China, while the other, the common persimmon, is native to the south-eastern United States.

Ripe persimmons are sweet fruits which soothe the digestive tract and help to relieve gastrointestinal inflammations such as enteritis. Persimmons contain diospyrol, an active ingredient found effective against parasitic infections, and in Thailand the fruit is used to expel worms. Unripe persimmons contain tannins and are astringent, which makes them beneficial in treating diarrhoea, dysentery, hypertension and coughs. However, it is important not to eat it in large quantities, certainly not more than one or two at a time, as it is known to cause intestinal blockage in some people.

PHENYLALANINE (PA), L-PHENYLALANINE

An essential amino acid which is abundant in meat and cheese, and without which the body cannot synthesize protein, PA has many important roles. It helps to form insulin, a hormone controlling blood sugar levels, and it is a precursor of tyrosine, which is needed by the thyroid gland to produce its hormone, thyroxine. PA is converted in the brain to epinephrine and norepinephrine, excitatory types of brain adrenalines which promote mental alertness, alleviate depression and suppress appetite very effectively, thus assisting in weight loss.

PA comes in two forms, L–phenylalanine (LPA) and D–phenylalanine (DPA), which are mirror images of each other: LPA has the nutritional value, while DPA has painkilling and depression–alleviating properties. A third form, DL–phenylalanine (DLPA) is both nutritional and therapeutic.

Studies have shown that DLPA can alleviate the pains of chronic conditions such as arthritis, lower back pain and headaches by protecting endorphins – the natural pain-blocking hormones secreted by the nerve cells.

Caution: Excessive doses of phenylalanine or DLPA can cause irritability, insomnia and elevated blood pressure. People with hypertension would do best to consult a nutritionist before taking DLPA. They should be started on a low dose (100 mg daily), which is then gradually increased while, at the same time, a check is kept on their blood pressure which should be monitored frequently.

Available at health food stores.

PHOSPHATIDYLSERINE (*PS*)

Phosphatidylserine is a relatively newly discovered nutrient which is normally produced by the brain. However, deficiencies of certain nutrients such as folic acid, vitamin B12 and essential fatty acid, can inhibit its production. PS is a vital phospholipid that maintains the integrity of brain cells, and its supplementation has been found to improve mental functions by increasing the levels of acetylcholine, which transmits brain messages. However, it is primarily used in the treatment of memory loss, depression, and behavioural and age-related brain changes in the elderly. Phosphatidylserine supplements, which are available in formulas in combination with other brain-enhancing nutrients, are becoming increasingly popular in health food shops.

PHOSPHORUS

Phosphorus is the second most abundant mineral in the body. It co-operates with **calcium** to ensure good bone mineralization and is present in every cell of the body. It is a constituent of DNA, the holder of our genetic blueprint, and of myelin, which insulates nerves. It is vital for the release of energy, converting **glucose** to glycogen (stored sugar) and helping to form **lecithin**. Phosphorus maintains strong bones and teeth, promotes growth and body repair, provides energy by helping to metabolize carbohydrates and fats, ensures proper functioning of nerves and maintains an acid–alkaline balance.

Phosphorus deficiencies are rare, but the mineral can be depleted by sugar and antacids, and deficiency symptoms include weak bones and teeth, rickets, gum infections, arthritis, loss of appetite and muscle weakness. Its best natural sources include meat, eggs, fish, whole grains, raw wheat germ, nuts and seeds. The normal daily requirement for adults is 800 mg, and for lactating women 1200 mg.

PHYTIC ACID

Phytic acid, or inositol hexaphosphate, is a form of **inositol**, one of the B vitamins. A component of the bran contained in grains, seeds and legumes, phytic acid binds with calcium, magnesium, iron, zinc and other minerals, preventing their absorption in the body. Thus, in order to prevent mineral deficiencies, it must be deactivated, and this can be done by bread-leavening, baking, or seed-sprouting.

Caution: Consumption of large quantities of raw bran can result in a deficiency of minerals such as calcium unless supplements of multi-mineral tablets are taken.

PINEAPPLES

Although pineapples are a rich source of vitamin C and potassium, they are low in other nutrients. However, they contain bromelain, a protein-splitting enzyme which increases digestion ability, and they can therefore be usefully eaten after a meat dish. Bromelain is also sold in capsules as a supplemental digestive aid. Pineapples are also diuretic and can be used to increase appetite, strengthen digestion, treat diarrhoea, destroy worms and reduce oedema.

Caution: Since unripe pineapples are acidic, they should not be eaten by anyone with a stomach or duodenal ulcer. Their acidity can also damage teeth.

PINE NUTS

Also known as pignolias, pine nuts are the seeds found in the cones of the pine tree, and in the past have been used as a staple food by both the Chinese and the American Indians. However, like many nuts, they are high in essential fatty acids and provide a poor source of protein.

Medicinally, pine nuts can be used to lubricate the intestines and soothe inflammations; they are also a mild laxative and helpful in treating dry cough.

Caution: Since pine nuts can quickly become rancid, they should be kept sealed in the refrigerator.

PLANTAIN SEE PSYLLIUM

PLUMS, PRUNES

Grown mainly in the temperate regions of the northern hemisphere, plums are high in potassium, and also contain moderate levels of calcium and iron. Due to their low fat content, they are a low-calorie food, and some of the golden varieties are a good source of beta carotene. Plums are diuretic and can be used in the treatment of liver conditions such as cirrhosis. Prunes are the dried fruit of a sweet variety of plum which is much richer in sugars, calcium and iron than standard plums. They contain a substance (dihydroxyphenyl isatin) which stimulates the bowels. Stewed prunes, or prune juice, have a laxative effect and are a traditional remedy for constipation.

POMEGRANATE

The fruit of a plant that is native to the warm climates of western Asia and north-western India, it is also grown commercially in the United States, particularly in the central regions of California. Pomegranates are a sweet-and-sour fruit, rich in iron and very astringent. Medicinally, they are mainly used to control diarrhoea and expel intestinal worms, but can also be helpful for treating bladder disturbances, strengthening gums and soothing mouth ulcers.

POPPY *(Papaver Somniferum)*

An annual herb, which is found wild in Asia and across Europe, it is noted for its brilliant red flowers. Although the seeds and oil of the plant have traditionally been used in cooking – particularly in cake making – the acute poisonous nature of the seeds should not be dismissed. When the unripe seed pods are crushed, they yield a milky juice that quickly hardens – and this is opium. Opium contains 25 different alkaloids, most of which are highly addictive; these include morphine, the well-known pain reliever, codeine and heroine.

Caution: Both the plant and its derivatives are poisonous and should only be used on prescription.

POTASSIUM

Potassium is a bulk mineral which constitutes 5 per cent of the total mineral content of the body. It is found mainly in intracellular fluids (i.e. fluids within cells), and has a multitude of functions. Together with sodium, potassium regulates the sodium–potassium balance which affects water retention and stimulates kidney function; it also promotes insulin secretion and is involved in nerve transmission and muscle contraction. In addition, potassium promotes the disposal of the body's wastes, increases mental alertness by increasing oxygen supply to the brain, reduces blood pressure, benefits diabetics by stimulating insulin production and helps digestion by stimulating stomach secretions.

Potassium deficiency symptoms include water retention (oedema), hypertension, irregular heartbeat, nervousness, fatigue and arthritis. Among the best natural sources of the mineral are citrus fruits, green leafy vegetables, bananas, potatoes, tomatoes and pineapples. Potassium deficiencies are rare, but can occur in cases of excessive diarrhoea or vomiting, or in the prolonged use of diuretics. In such cases, potassium supplements are necessary, and they are also sometimes recommended for diabetics, in order to improve their insulin sensitivity. No daily requirements are set for potassium, but an average daily consumption for adults of between 1.9 g and 5.6 g is considered normal.

POTATO

A member of the nightshade family, Solanaceae, the potato is a native of South America and was first introduced into Europe in the mid-sixteenth century. Nowadays, it is the world's most widely grown vegetable and one of its most important foods. Potatoes have a high nutritional value and are grown in most countries. They are a highly starchy food and, when eaten with the skin, or peel, a good source of vegetable protein, potassium, vitamin C, iron, phosphorus, niacin and enzymes – although old potatoes are low in vitamin C. Medicinally, potatoes can help to relieve arthritis and reduce water retention due to their high potassium content. They also neutralize body acids and potato juice can be used to treat stomach and duodenal ulcers. The fresh juice is sometimes used to reduce hypertension, and promote intestinal flora.

PREGNENOLONE

A recently highlighted natural hormone (also known as preg), it is formed from cholesterol in the organs that produce steroid hormones, such as the adrenal glands, and is a precursor of **DHEA**. Apart from its conversion to DHEA or progesterone, preg has also been claimed to improve energy, enhance mental acuity, regulate mood disorders and relieve fatigue. In addition, it is reputed to improve memory and learning capabilities. It is currently used mainly for its benefits in chronic conditions such as arthritis, psoriasis and pre-menstrual syndrome. However, although pregnenolone is now being sold over the counter in the US, it should be used with caution since, to date, relatively little research has been done on it.

PRESERVATIVES

Preservatives are additives, usually chemicals such as nitrates and phosphates, which are added during the processing of food to prevent spoilage and reduce food poisoning risks by inhibiting the growth of bacteria, viruses and fungi. Nowadays, a wide range of foods are commercially preserved, from soft drinks, jams and cheeses, to beer, wine and meats. Some of the most popular preservatives, such as benzoic acid, benzoates, sulphur dioxide, and particularly sulphites, have been reported to trigger allergic reactions such as asthma in susceptible people.

PROANTHOCYANIDINS see BIOFLAVONOIDS

PROBIOTICS

This is a general descriptive name for all products which regenerate the intestines and rejuvenate the whole body. Probiotics enhance the growth of intestinal flora – the friendly bacteria in the intestines – while reducing disease-causing bacteria. In general, they promote healthy biological systems, as opposed to **antibiotics** and contraceptive pills which do the opposite, promoting decaying processes in the gut. Probiotics include **yogurts**, buttermilk and other sour milks, digestive **enzymes**, **FOS**, and fermented foods such as **sauerkraut**, **miso** and **tofu**. Yogurts and sour milks contain cultures of friendly bacteria, including **Lactobacillus acidolhilus**, Lactobacillus bulgaricus, Bifidobacteria longum and Streptococcus thermophilus, which are usually listed on the food labels. When consumed regularly, these friendly bacteria are highly beneficial to the body. They assist food absorption, increase the production of vitamins, maintain proper acidity in the intestines, increase resistance against disease and prevent the development of colon cancer and thrush (candida). FOS are types of sugars which feed selectively only the friendly bacteria and enhance their growth. Overgrowth of pathogenic bacteria in the intestines is associated with conditions such as allergies, eczema, bad breath, constipation, arthritis, headaches, sinus congestion, high cholesterol, colitis, candida, yeast infection and cystitis.

PROLINE, L-PROLINE

One of the non–essential amino acids, proline supplements are recommended in the treatment of short-term depression. They are claimed to give many people a sense of relief and happiness. Proline is also involved in the production of collagen and can therefore improve skin texture. Available at health food stores and as formulas.

PROPOLIS

Hailed as a natural antibiotic with no side effects, propolis is a resinous substance collected by bees from plants and trees (mainly poplar), waxes, essential oils and pollen, which are all mixed by the bee's salivary glands and used in the construction of the hive. It has been used for thousands of years for a wide range of conditions and its name, which signifies its protective effects, comes from the Greek 'pro' meaning 'before' and 'polis' meaning 'city', i.e. 'defence before the city'.

Propolis contains a great variety of amino acids, vitamins, minerals and bioflavonoids and, in the same way that it is used by the bees as a sticky filler to seal and protect the hive, propolis can be used for similar beneficial effects on the human body. For instance, the Greeks used it to treat wounds and Hippocrates himself, the father of modern medicine, prescribed propolis for sores and ulcers.

During the past twenty years, scientific studies have 'rediscovered' propolis and found it to be a great booster of the immune system, enhancing the immune response and resistance against disease by stimulating the formation of immune cells. A recent study at Oxford University has revealed that propolis can help to cure inflammations, while Chinese research has found propolis effective in treating hypertension and arteriosclerosis, and Soviet scientists have shown that propolis can prevent ulcers. In fact, propolis is now increasingly used to treat conditions as wide-ranging as colds, sore throats, coughs, allergies, vaginal infections, painful menstruation, acne and herpes.

When buying propolis it is important to check on the quantity included in each capsule. The recommended dosage is 1.5–3 g per day, which should be taken on an empty stomach, preferably first thing in the morning or at bedtime.

PROSTAGLANDINS SEE EVENING PRIMROSE OIL (EPO); FATS

PROTEIN

As a macronutrient, protein is the most plentiful component of the body, after water. It not only builds up body structures such as cells, tissues and skeleton, but also creates the body's functional factors, such as hormones, antibodies, DNA and digestive secretions. Protein enables children's growth, and is equally important in adulthood, when growth has ceased, to supply 'spare parts' to counteract the wear and tear of daily living. Various proteins, such as those in red blood cells, hormones and immune cells, are constantly being broken down and need to be rebuilt. Proteins also serve as a source of energy and heat, providing 4 calories per gram. Their richest dietary sources are animal foods such as eggs, meat, fish and dairy products.

Protein is made up of amino acids, in the same way that a wall is composed of bricks, and during the digestion process, it is broken down in the body to its basic 'bricks', the amino acids, which are then absorbed into the bloodstream and reassembled for new protein synthesis. Twenty-two amino acids are linked together in various forms to create the many and varied types of proteins, such as hair, bone or nails, and these processes are supervised by the nucleic acids RNA and DNA, the specific proteins which contain our genetic blueprint. Eight of these amino acids, which cannot be produced by the body and must be supplied by food, are classified as 'essential amino acids', namely: leucine, isoleucine, valine, methionine, threonine, lysine, phenylalanine and tryptophan.

An adequate supply of dietary protein is of utmost importance in order to maintain optimal health, growth, function and rejuvenation of the body. Symptoms of protein deficiency are many and varied, ranging from falling hair, brittle nails and rough skin, to fatigue, anaemia and low sexual drive. In addition to creating protein, various amino acids, both essential and non–essential, have been found to have specific beneficial effects on health, and these amino acids are available as nutritional supplements.

PSYLLIUM, PLANTAIN
(Plantago Ovata, Plantago Major)

Psyllium is a perennial herb which is mainly cultivated in Asia. The seeds are rich both in mucilaginous substances and fibre. The leaves of P. major, the greater or common plantain, which grows prolifically as a weed throughout the British Isles, also contain tannins. Psyllium is an intestinal lubricant that soothes the digestive tract and is beneficial in cases of internal infections, ulcers and diverticulosis. It is also an astringent and its decoctions, which promote blood–clotting, are used on wounds and haemorrhoids. However, its most common use is in fighting constipation. Mixed with water, the powdered seeds make an excellent laxative as, like bran, they absorb water in the intestine and swell, stimulating a natural bowel movement. Psyllium husk powder in bulk and capsule form is available in health food shops.

PULSES SEE LEGUMES

PUMPKIN

Pumpkin is a sweet vegetable which probably originated in North America, where it is still widely grown and eaten. It provides a good source of beta carotene, calcium, iron and some B vitamins. it can also help to regulate blood sugar levels, and is thus of benefit to hypoglycaemics. Pumpkin promotes the expulsion of mucus from the throat, bronchi and lungs and its regular use is said to benefit bronchial asthma. Pumpkin seeds are rich in zinc, and are known for their ability to destroy parasitic intestinal worms, both in children and adults.

PYCNOGENOL

Pycnogenol is the trade name for a group of **bioflavonoids** called proanthocyanidins. Although these flavonoids can be extracted from various foods such as fruits, grains, vegetables and grape seeds, pycnogenol is derived under patent, from the French maritime pine tree (Pinus maritima).

The proanthocyanidins in pycnogenol are powerful **antioxidants** and free radical scavengers. In this respect, pycnogenol is a supernutrient supplement. It has been found to be fifty times better than **vitamin E** and twenty times better than **vitamin C** in scavenging free radicals. Pycnogenol has anti–ageing properties and is usually taken to boost immune response and prevent the degenerative diseases of ageing, such as cancer, atherosclerosis, heart attack, arthritis and diabetes.

PYRIDOXINE SEE VITAMIN B6

Q

QUERCETIN

A **bioflavonoid**, which is becoming increasingly popular, quercetin serves as a backbone for other flavonoids and is considered to be the most active of them all. Quercetin has a wide range of beneficial effects. It has been found to be a powerful **antioxidant**, neutralizes free radicals, which are the underlying causes of the degenerative diseases of ageing such as heart disease, cancer and arthritis; it has also been reported to possess strong and prolonged anti-inflammatory and wound-healing properties. In addition, it is reported to be effective against viruses, especially oral herpes.

Quercetin has also been shown to have anti-cancer properties and studies have revealed that it can inhibit the proliferation of malignant cells in breast and ovarian cancers and leukaemia. It has also been found to inhibit histamine release, making it useful in the treatment of allergies. Additional studies have reported on the ability of quercetin to delay the onset of cataract, and, since it is able to enhance insulin secretion, it is also useful in the control of diabetes.

Quercetin is abundant in fruits and vegetables such as citrus rind, garlic, onions and blue-green algae and supplements of quercetin are now available in health food shops in capsule form.

Caution: High doses of quercetin supplements may cause diarrhoea.

QUINOA

A grain, which thrives in the high, cold altitudes of the Andes Mountains of South America, where it has been grown for thousands of years, it was one of the staple foods of the Aztecs and known as the 'mother grain'.

The protein content of quinoa is the highest of any of the grains, both in quantity and in quality. It also contains more fat than other grains, and has more calcium than milk. In addition, it is a very good source of iron, B vitamins, vitamin E and phosphorus. The grain is still cultivated in the Andes, and remains one of the chief foods of Andean Indians. It is also exported to the US, where it is processed and marketed as grain, flour or pasta. Quinoa can be cooked in the same way as other grains, such as rice; it is also included in breakfast cereals.

R

RADISH *(Raphanus Sativus)*

An annual plant, which is cultivated for its succulent tubers, radish is eaten raw and mainly used in salads. It is an astringent and diuretic, and is used to promote bile flow.

Radishes, and their juice, are an old home remedy for coughs, rheumatism and gall bladder problems. The leaves of the plant, which are usually discarded, are very nutritious, containing almost ten times as much vitamin C as the roots. They are also rich in calcium, iron, sodium, phosphorus, sulphur and potassium. In Yemenite folk medicine, radishes are used to eliminate kidney stones. Half a cup of fresh radish juice each morning on an empty stomach usually dissolves even the most stubborn stones, passing them out of the body in the urine.

Caution: Large kidney stones can scratch the urinary passage and cause bleeding as they are passed out. Two tablespoonfuls of olive oil can supply lubrication and ease the elimination. Radishes are not recommended for people with gastrointestinal inflammations or ulcers.

RASPBERRY *(Rubus Idaeus)*

A widespread shrubby plant which grows wild, raspberry is cultivated for its red berries. It is an effective astringent and the leaves are rich in vitamins, minerals and fragarine, a substance which prevents uterine contractions. Infusion of the leaves can be used to prevent premature birth and painful menstruation. Fresh raspberry juice is an excellent cooling beverage for fevers.

Raspberry leaf tea, which is available from health food stores as tea bags, can be used to stop diarrhoea, treat stomach and intestinal ulcers, and help with the healing of wounds. It is also used as a gargle.

RAW JUICE FASTING SEE FASTING

RDA (RECOMMENDED DAILY ALLOWANCES)

These are the amounts of vitamins and minerals required on a daily basis by the average adult. The RDA values have been created by calculating the amounts of nutrients in average diets and then adding a 'margin of safety'. However, RDA values tend to be set extremely low and have been challenged by many nutritional authorities, especially as RDAs represent average amounts for populations, rather than individuals, and people are biochemically very different from each other. For example, some people burn vitamins quicker than others, and some may have absorption defects of certain nutrients and therefore need an additional intake of these nutrients.

Initially, RDAs were intended to prevent nutrient deficiencies, but today the major public trend is towards optimal nutrition, which provides an optimal feeling of well-being and an optimal lifespan. This is the reason why many people use nutritional supplements, sometimes supplementing their diets many times above the RDA levels.

REISHI *(Ganoderma Lucidum)*

This is an exceptional Chinese **mushroom** that has long been highly rated in traditional Chinese medicine as a cure-all and has been used in the treatment of a variety of disorders. It is believed to promote health and longevity and to be the best booster of the body's immunity against diseases. Reishi contains **germanium** and is considered to have a powerful effect against tumours and cancers. Recent research has found reishi to be beneficial in relieving fatigue and stress, treating viral infections and joint inflammations, lowering high cholesterol and triglycerides, reducing heart disease symptoms, regenerating the liver, alleviating allergies, calming the nervous system, helping with the treatment of diabetes and reducing the side effects of chemotherapy. Reishi mushrooms (available from health food stores as capsules) are now increasingly incorporated as an ingredient in many multivitamin–mineral supplements.

RENNIN *(Chymosin)*

Rennin, or chymosin, is a protein–splitting enzyme which is used to coagulate milk in the making of cheese. It is contained in rennet, a substance which is found in the lining of calves' stomachs. Rennin is used to make the milk separate into curds and whey. The curds are then pressed to drain off the whey and, at this point, they form a soft cheese, such as cottage cheese; otherwise, they are allowed to mature to form the harder cheeses.

RETINOL

Retinol is the fat-soluble, absorbable form of **vitamin A** which is only present in animal food (especially liver), meat, fish, dairy foods and eggs. It is thought to serve as a precursor to two active forms of vitamin A, retinal and retinoic acid. Retinal is mainly involved with improving vision and reproduction, while retinoic acid performs the other duties of vitamin A, such as proper growth and skin health. Ninety per cent of the body's retinol is stored in the liver.

The vegetable form of vitamin A, beta carotene or provitamin A, cannot be used as such and must first be converted in the body to retinol.

RHUBARB *(RHEUM PALMATUM)*

A perennial vegetable that grows wild in China, it is used mainly for its roots and rhizomes. As an appetite stimulant and astringent, rhubarb is effective for both constipation and diarrhoea, depending on the amounts used. Large amounts can promote diarrhoea while tiny amounts will have a constipative effect.

Caution: The leaves are high in oxalic acid, which in itself can be poisonous; it can also bind with calcium to form insoluble crystals, which are the precursors of kidney stones, and people with a tendency to kidney stones or gravel should avoid rhubarb.

RIBOFLAVIN SEE VITAMIN B2

RNA SEE **NUCLEIC ACIDS**

RICE

Rice is a cereal grain which is one of the world's most important food crops. It forms the main diet of more than half of the world's population, most of whom live in Asia, where the grain is thought to have originated. It thrives in the warm, wet climates of tropical areas and is available in several types and shapes. Natural rice is a rich source of the B vitamins, vitamin E, fibre and unsaturated fatty acids, but unfortunately refining removes most of these nutrients – whole grain brown rice is both nutritious and easily digestible, while white rice is nutritionally inferior.

Rice is the least allergenic of the cereal grains and is well tolerated even by infants and people with digestive disorders. It provides a good home remedy for diarrhoea, nausea and diabetes. Its B vitamins nourish the nervous system and help to relieve depression; it is also used by coeliacs because it does not contain gluten.

Short grain rice has a nuttier flavour and a thicker consistency and is better for nervousness than the long grain, which is less sticky. Basmati rice is slightly aromatic and lighter in texture than other varieties, making it more suitable for the overweight. Wild rice, which is known to benefit the kidneys and bladder, is a grass native to North America and is more related to corn than to rice.

Rice can also be sprouted and used for people with weak digestion and poor appetite. (see *SPROUTS*)

ROSE, ROSEHIPS *(ROSA SPP.)*

Although one of the most highly cultivated of flowers, the delicate pink blooms of the wild rose are still widely found adorning roadside hedges in early summer. As prickly shrubs, roses come in a great variety of species and have been used for therapeutic purposes for many centuries. Traditionally, a tea of dried rose petals can be used for headaches and dizziness, while a decoction of the petals may help mouth sores. The rosehips of the wild rose are very high in vitamin C and are used for making tisanes, syrups and vitamin C supplements. They are mildly laxative and are also useful as nerve tonics. The hips, like the petals, can be used to treat headaches and dizziness, clear mouth sores and as a mouthwash; they can also be used to purify the blood.

ROSEMARY *(ROSMARINUS OFFICINALIS)*

A beautiful, fragrant evergreen shrub which is native to the Mediterranean regions, it has a variety of herbal uses. An infusion of the leaves and flowering tops is a sedative which can be used to relieve flatulence and headaches, promote perspiration, increase bile flow and stimulate menstruation. Rosemary leaves are used as a culinary seasoning and to make essential oils for aromatherapy. They are also used externally, mainly in shampoos and other hair preparations.

ROYAL JELLY

A bee product, royal jelly is a thick milky substance that is produced by young nurse bees from pollen and honey. It is the food that converts a regular 'worker' bee to a 'queen' bee, who is then able to lay eggs and reproduce. Royal jelly contains the B vitamins, and is particularly rich in pantothenic acid, the B vitamin that relieves stress and promotes fertility and healthy reproduction. Royal jelly also contains vitamins A, C, D and E, together with minerals, hormones, a vast number of amino acids, and antibiotic and antibacterial components, not all of which are isolated.

Royal jelly is known to strengthen the immune system and to help in such conditions as fatigue, low sex drive, liver disease, stomach ulcers, kidney disease and skin problems. Royal jelly spoils easily, and is therefore usually sold blended with **honey**, or in capsules. It is best kept refrigerated and taken on an empty stomach.

RUE *(RUTA GRAVEOLENS)*

An aromatic, perennial plant native to the Mediterranean countries, it is also widely cultivated elsewhere. The aromatic leaves are high in rutin, the bioflavonoid that strengthens capillaries and blood vessels. An infusion of the leaves is diuretic, slightly increases the blood pressure and has an abortifacient effect (inducing abortion). In Yemenite folk medicine, rue is used to treat nervous breakdowns and to stimulate the onset of delayed menstruation.

Caution: Rue must not be taken during pregnancy. Available from specialist ethnic grocers and herbalists.

RUTIN

Rutin is a crystalline glucoside, a **bioflavonoid** closely related to hesperidin. It is present in many plants but its richest source is **buckwheat**. Rutin strengthens fragile capillaries and blood vessels, inhibits internal haemorrhages, reduces blood pressure and increases blood circulation to the hands and feet. It is also used in the treatment of piles. Rutin is an antioxidant and can help to prevent radiation damage: its action is greatly increased when combined with **vitamin C**. Rutin is available in capsules as a supplement.

RYE

A cereal grain which is widely grown in the cool climates of northern Europe, Asia, and North America, it formed the major ingredient in the bread eaten in medieval Europe. Rye is a very nourishing hard grain, regarded by many as nutritionally superior to wheat. It is high in protein, calcium and iron, and a good source of vitamins B1, B2 and niacin. Rye bread increases strength and stamina, cleans arteries, prevents anaemia, and aids the growth of hair and nails. Rich in fluorine, rye sprouts or soaked rye flakes can strengthen teeth enamel and help bone formation. Rye flour is ideally suited to making sourdough bread. Widely available.

S

SAFFLOWER SEED AND OIL

Safflower is an annual grain cultivated in the USA and Europe. A tea made from the flowers is diuretic and increases perspiration. Of all the kitchen oils, safflower oil is highest in polyunsaturated fatty acids. Its 79 per cent polyunsaturates, which contain the essential linoleic and linolenic acids, are known to lower cholesterol levels and prevent heart attacks and strokes. However, this is only a nutritional asset when the oil is fresh, because the higher its content of unsaturates, the more vulnerable an oil is to oxidation and rancidity and, once rancid, the unsaturated fatty acids are converted to irritating substances. Widely available.

SAFFRON *(Crocus Sativus)*

A small perennial plant cultivated in many parts of the world, including Europe and Asia, saffron is both an expensive aromatic spice and a medical herb with several benefits. Traditionally, its flower stigmas are a well-known aphrodisiac. Saffron is also believed to strengthen the appetite, soothe the alimentary canal, increase bile flow, clear liver stagnancy, help menopausal difficulties and relieve phlegm. In small doses, saffron has been used to treat coughs, bloated stomach, colic and insomnia, and it is sometimes used in herb liqueurs as an appetite stimulant. Widely available.

Caution: Saffron contains a poison which can damage the kidneys and nerves and 10 g can provide a fatal dose for humans. It should therefore be used in small amounts only.

SAGE *(SALVIA OFFICINALIS)*

A perennial shrub which grows wild in the Mediterranean regions, the herb is also widely cultivated for its culinary and medicinal properties. It has an ancient reputation of 'warding off evils', and its leaves are used both in infusions and as a culinary seasoning. Sage tea is astringent, sedative and expels gas; it clears the respiratory tract, makes a good gargle for sore throats and helps overcome colds. Sage is useful for night sweats as it reduces sweating. It also reduces milk flow in nursing mothers prior to weaning, prevents the formation of kidney stones by dissolving residues of uric acid, and regularizes menstruation. An infusion of sage can be applied to the scalp to reduce dandruff. Widely available.

SALMON

The salmon is a fish with the least saturated fat and cholesterol. It contains a valuable source of the highly beneficial omega-3 fatty acids, EPA and DHA. These essential fatty acids are effective in preventing serious cardiovascular conditions, such as hardening of the arteries, blood clots, hypertension, high cholesterol levels, heart attacks and strokes.

SALMONELLA

Salmonella is a bacteria which can be found in spoiled foods, raw eggs, unpasteurized milk, and also in the intestines of animals. It is the most common cause of food poisoning and is mainly contracted from contaminated foods, particularly eggs, chicken and meat products – poorly cooked meats are a great risk. It is also easily transmitted by unhygienic food preparation, storing and handling and unclean cutlery or cooking utensils. The effects of salmonella poisoning can vary in severity, ranging from diarrhoea, cramps and vomiting, to fever and infections, and these can sometimes be fatal, particularly in those whose immune system is weak, such as infants and the elderly.

SALT *(Sodium Chloride)*

The richest contributor of sodium in the average diet, table or culinary salt has been indiscriminately condemned as a risky food, leaving many people confused about its use. It should be remembered, however, that in the right amounts, sodium is a much needed mineral in the body. For example, it stimulates kidneys and also gastric juices, enabling proper digestion; it promotes sweating and energy, helps to maintain a proper acid–alkaline balance and assists the transmission of nerve messages (see SODIUM).

Salt has been incriminated for increasing water retention and elevating blood pressure. Until recently, people who were overweight or hypertensive, and those with heart conditions, were warned to avoid salt and many were put on sodium-free diets. However, a new study of thousands of hypertensive patients has shown that reducing salt intake is unnecessary, unless people are aged over 45 and suffer from high blood pressure. Lowering the salt intake of younger people, even with hypertension, has been found to be of limited value. The study recommends instead that patients should take more exercise and drink less alcohol. The harmful effects of severe salt restriction on a large scale are only now becoming appreciated.

SALTBUSH *(ARTIPLEX HALIMUS)*

This is a bush that grows in desert areas such as the dry grazing areas of southern Australia and around the shores of the Mediterranean Sea. Its leaves are rich in minerals, especially salt, and in fact the leaves actually taste salty when chewed. Two of the minerals contained in its leaves, chromium and manganese, have been found to be very beneficial in the treatment of diabetes, and have even been reported to produce a cure in some of the milder cases. Available from specialist ethnic grocers.

SARSAPARILLA *(SMILAX OFFICINALIS)*

A tropical perennial plant, which is found wild in South America, its root is used to make root beer, a popular beverage in North America, particularly in the American Midwest. A tea prepared from the root has both tonic and diuretic properties, and is used to expel gas and increase perspiration. It is also said to help in the treatment of colds, fevers, gout and rheumatism. In Spanish folk medicine, sarsaparilla was claimed to have a regenerative effect on the genital organs, and was used to help the treatment of venereal diseases such as syphilis and gonorrhoea. Available from health food stores, herbalists and as formulas.

SASSAFRAS *(SASSAFRAS ALBIDUM)*

A tree of the laurel family, it grows wild in the eastern and Pacific north-west regions of the USA. A tea prepared from the bark is a strong stimulant and was used by the American Indians as an aphrodisiac. An infusion promotes perspiration and urination, purifies the blood, and is used in conditions such as gout, rheumatism and arthritis. Sassafras tea was once popular as a tonic drink. Available from larger health food stores and herbalists.

SAUERKRAUT

A healthy **probiotic** food, sauerkraut is made by fermenting (pickling) cabbage, with or without salt. It is easily made at home by crushing raw cabbage and storing it in a ceramic pot or glass container for about a week. Cabbage can be combined with a variety of herbs and vegetables, such as garlic, carrots or seaweeds, to produce different types of sauerkraut, which can be stored in the refrigerator for several months, although the salted variety has a longer storage life.

Sauerkraut can regenerate the intestines and rejuvenate the body by increasing the intestinal flora; it balances stomach secretions, and improves digestion. Saltless sauerkraut helps to maintain a correct acid–alkali balance, strengthen the immune system, improve resistance to disease, stimulate blood formation and increase energy and well-being. For best results, sauerkraut should be eaten on a daily basis by adding a small amount to meals.

SAW PALMETTO (SERENOA SERRULATA)

A small palm tree which grows wild in coastal regions of North America, it is also known as 'dwarf palm'. Saw palmetto was traditionally used as a food by the south–eastern American Indians, and it has recently made headlines in the media as a treatment for enlarged prostate in men.

The therapeutic value of saw palmetto lies in its berries, which contain an unusual mix of fatty acids, phytosterols and alcohols that has been found to have a beneficial effect on the size and health of the prostate. This is a muscular gland that surrounds the urethra of males at the base of the bladder and it becomes enlarged when its cells reproduce quicker than normal as a result of over-secretion of hormones. This can be due to age-related changes, so that enlargement of the prostate gland can be a potential problem for any man over 50. Enlargement of the prostate can produce several uncomfortable symptoms such as difficult or frequent urination, interrupted sleep patterns due to frequent night-time visits to the bathroom, or incomplete emptying of the bladder. In extreme cases, the prostate can develop inflammation or cancer.

Saw palmetto berries have been found to inhibit the hormonal secretion of the prostate and relieve much of the discomfort. Saw palmetto extracts are available in capsule form at health food shops. The normal recommended dose is 160 mg, taken once or twice daily.

SEAWEEDS

Seaweeds, or marine algae, is a general descriptive name for sea vegetables. They are extremely rich in iodine and in other minerals, such as calcium, iron, and fluorine, and have been known for centuries for their ability to promote health. They are especially beneficial to thyroid function, and can also lower cholesterol, alkalize the blood, remove radioactivity residues, help with weight loss and are important in bone mineralization and density. Seaweeds are used to treat conditions such as goitre, water retention (oedema) and swollen lymph glands. They come in several colours – brown, red, green, blue-green and yellow-green – each of which has its own individual properties in addition to the common properties of the plant. The most commonly used seaweeds include **kelp**, **agar**, dulse, hijiki, **kombu**, arame, wakame, **nori** and **Irish moss**.

SELENIUM

Selenium is a trace element that works best when combined with **vitamin E**. It is needed by the body to form glutathione peroxidase, an important **antioxidant** enzyme which protects the body from the damaging effects of free radicals and prevents the degenerative diseases of ageing. In fact, selenium deficiency is a known factor in premature ageing, heart attacks and cancer, and it has been estimated that if the majority of people took selenium supplements, the incidence of cancer could be reduced by 70 per cent! In conjunction with vitamin E, selenium helps the body to eliminate toxic elements such as lead, cadmium and mercury.

The beneficial effects of selenium are many and varied. It increases immunity to diseases, slows down ageing, alleviates menopausal discomfort, promotes energy and sexual potency, and helps to prevent auto-immune diseases such as arthritis and multiple sclerosis and degenerative diseases such as cancer and atherosclerosis.

Some of the deficiency symptoms of selenium are manifested as fatigue, susceptibility to infections, premature ageing, predisposition to cancer and low sexual potency – selenium is concentrated in the male sex glands and is lost in ejaculated semen. Dietary sources of selenium are limited as plants do not require selenium for growth and can happily prosper in selenium-poor soils. Among the best natural sources are brewer's yeast, raw wheat germ, tuna, onions, nuts and seeds. An average daily consumption for adults of between 50 and 200 mcg is recommended, with a range of 50–80 mcg for children. Selenium is available as a supplement in health food shops.

SENNA (CASSIA ACUTIFOLIA)

The dried pods and leaves of the cassia tree, which grows wild in North African countries, senna contains two active glycosides and is a well-known remedy for chronic constipation. An infusion of the leaves and pods will act as a strong laxative. Senna is often combined with other substances to eliminate intestinal worms; it can also help to counteract bad breath. Available from health food stores and widely incorporated in laxative formulas.

Caution: Senna should not be used in case of haemorrhoids.

SERINE SEE PHOSPHATIDYLSERINE (PS)

SEROTONIN

Serotonin has recently been receiving considerable media attention for its many beneficial effects. It is one of the neurotransmitters, i.e. brain chemicals that carry messages between the nerve cells, and unlike other excitatory neurotransmitters, such as adrenalin, serotonin is an inhibiting or calming neurotransmitter and reduces brain cell activity. It counteracts depression, anxiety and fear, lifting the spirits; it also increases libido, induces sleep, improves memory and concentration, dampens the appetite and aids weight reduction. In fact, drugs which raise serotonin levels are now being used to help with weight loss.

Unfortunately, serotonin cannot be taken as a supplement because it is broken down during digestion. It is derived in the body from the amino acid **tryptophan** which is abundant in foods such as milk and bananas. Starchy foods such as potatoes can also help to raise serotonin levels by increasing insulin which, in turn, raises tryptophan levels.

SESAME SEEDS

A annual herb which originated in Africa or India, it is now widely cultivated in the tropical regions of China, India, Japan, Mexico and the south-western states of the United States.

Sesame seeds are very nutritious and provide an excellent source of protein, calcium, unsaturated fatty acids, magnesium, vitamins A, E and niacin. Available hulled or unhulled, the unhulled seeds – as used in breads or grain dishes – are more nutritious because most of the mineral content of the seed is contained in the hull. Hulled sesame seeds are commonly available as sesame butter, called tahini, which can be used in a number of ways. Combined with honey, tahini makes delicious spreads; blended with water, lemon and garlic, it provides a base for a healthy salad dressing which is very popular in the Middle East. Allowed to stand for a while, the oil separates from tahini and can be used as an excellent cooking oil; it can also be used externally to soothe skin problems. Tahini can be combined with water to prepare sesame milk, which is used to lubricate the intestines, help to relieve constipation, and is also recommended for stiff joints, weak knees, nervous spasms and increasing milk secretion in nursing mothers.

SHEPHERD'S PURSE (CAPSELLA BURSA-PASTORIS)

An annual herb which is widespread, growing wild throughout Europe, particularly in poor soils and wastelands, it is rich in calcium, sodium, and vitamins C and K. The whole plant has medicinal properties and is an effective blood coagulant, which can be used to stop bleeding, both external and internal, including excessive menstrual bleeding. It is also a diuretic. Available from health food stores and incorporated in nutritional formulas.

SHORT-CHAIN FATTY ACIDS (SCFA)

SCFAs are produced naturally in the intestines from dietary fibre by the intestinal flora. The three SCFAs, acetic acid, propionic acid and butyric acid, have important functions. Acetate and propionate are stored in the liver and used for energy production. Butyrate is an important energy source for the metabolic activity of the colon. It has effective anti-cancer effects and is thought to be responsible for the cancer-inhibiting properties of dietary fibre. Butyrate is also used in enemas in the treatment of ulcerative colitis. Different fibres produce differing amounts of SCFAs in the colon. Pectins (from apples), guar gum and legume fibres produce more SCFAs than oat bran or corn fibre.

SILICON

Although, as a constituent of sand and rocks, silicon is the most abundant element contained in the earth's crust, in the human body it is found in only trace amounts as silica (silicon dioxide). In spite of this small overall amount, however, silica is present in almost every tissue of the body and is essential for cell growth. It is especially concentrated in the hair, nails and connective tissues such as the skin. It can inhibit the greying of hair, keep the skin smooth and supple and prevent brittle nails. For these reasons, it is incorporated into many cosmetic formulas. However, a distinction should be made between water-soluble silica and the controversial silicone breast implants. Despite the similarity in the name, natural silica differs considerably from breast implant silicone, which is an industrial polymer containing controversial hydrocarbons suspected of being carcinogenic.

Silica and silica gel have been reported to be beneficial in treating many disorders, including heartburn, ulcers, gastritis, colitis, varicose veins, bronchitis, arteriosclerosis, gum recession, allergic rashes and many others.

The best natural sources of silica include horsetail herb, oats, millet, barley, onions, whole wheat and red beet. Silica supplements, both for internal and external use, are available from health food shops in many forms, such as effervescent or chewable tablets, capsules, powders and silica gel. All come with directions for use.

SLIPPERY ELM SEE ELM

SOD *(SUPEROXIDE DISMUTASE)*

This very important antioxidant enzyme, which includes copper and zinc, is found naturally within cells. It protects cells and tissues from the damage of superoxide free radicals and is a general anti-ageing enzyme. It is reported to be especially helpful in preventing the damage to joints, membranes and lubricating fluids which occurs in rheumatoid arthritis. It also helps to prevent cataracts.

SOD is available as a supplement although, when taken orally, it is mostly destroyed in the digestive tract. However, when administered in injections, it is reported to have been beneficial for both osteoarthritis and rheumatoid arthritis.

SODIUM

The main component of salt is sodium, a mineral prevalent in the body which is found mainly in the fluids surrounding body cells, rather than within them. Sodium is highly important in maintaining osmotic pressure in tissues, enabling oxygen and nutrients to move in or out of cells; it stimulates the kidneys and keeps calcium soluble, preventing kidney stones; it also stimulates the secretion of gastric juices, helping digestion, promotes sweating and helps to prevent heat strokes, and improves feelings of lassitude in people with low blood pressure. Together with potassium, it participates in nerve transmissions and maintains a correct acid–alkaline balance.

Excessive sodium tends to elevate blood pressure, constrict blood vessels and cause water retention, resulting in oedema and hypertension. People with high blood pressure, heart disease, oedema, or those who are overweight, are usually advised to avoid salt and use low-sodium diets. This can be done by using potassium–based salt substitutes, as well as herb powders such as celery, basil, caraway, mustard or parsley.

Deficiencies of salt are very uncommon, but can occur as a result of excessive perspiration. Some of the best natural sources include table salt, kelp and seaweeds, meats, beets, carrots, chard and dandelion greens.

Caution: Excessive sodium intake should be balanced by increased potassium, since sodium causes the excretion of potassium in the urine.

SORBITOL

Sorbitol is a type of sugar, which is commercially refined from glucose and sucrose. It is about 60 per cent as sweet as sugar and is popular among diabetics since it does not raise insulin levels as sharply as table sugar. Most of the sorbitol is converted in the body to carbon dioxide and fructose, with only a small part of it being converted to glucose; this is then absorbed through the intestines over a relatively long period of time so that a sharp insulin release is not triggered as is the case with table sugar. Since insulin is known to promote detrimental changes in the cardiovascular system, sorbitol is therefore a much more desirable sweetener than ordinary sugar, even for healthy people. In addition, the slow metabolism of sorbitol does not tax the sugar-balancing glands and causes much less tooth decay. Sorbitol also increases the absorption of certain vitamins, such as B12, which is why it is included in many multivitamin tablets.

SOYBEAN

An ancient staple crop of Asia, the soybean is a legume noted for its high vegetable protein content (38 per cent), which is greater than the protein content of milk. The crop has long been considered a solution to famine in Asia, since an acre of soybeans produces 20 times more usable protein than the same acreage used for grazing beef or growing fodder.

In recent years, soybeans have developed into one of the world's major sources of vegetable oil and texturized vegetable protein (TVP) and, as such, they are included in many foods, including ice cream, soy sauce, beansprouts and **tofu**. Soya milk does not contain the saturated fat, cholesterol and toxic residues of dairy milk. It has, to a large extent, replaced dairy milk in many people's diets and revolutionized their eating habits.

Soybeans have been found to be a storehouse of phytochemicals – beneficial antioxidant nutrients, such as saponins, phytosterols and phenolic acids – which protect the body from free radical damage, reducing the risk of the degenerative diseases of ageing, such as heart attack, cancer and strokes. Two of the best anticarcinogens in soya are some plant oestrogens, which prevent breast cancer, and genistein, which inhibits the growth of cancer cells. Soybeans have also been found to be beneficial in reducing cholesterol levels and preventing heart attacks. Research has shown that the substitution of soya products in the daily diet for just part of the normal meat and dairy milk intake can provide a number of health benefits.

All widely available. (See also SPROUTS)

SPINACH

A popular garden vegetables which is native to south-east
Asia, spinach is an excellent source of iron, calcium, chlorophyll, beta carotene (provitamin A), vitamin C, riboflavin,
sodium and potassium. It is a diuretic and laxative, and can
also be used to stop minor haemorrhaging such as nosebleeds. As it is rich in iron and chlorophyll, spinach builds
the blood, while its sulphur content helps to clean the liver
and relieve herpes irritations. In addition, its vitamin A content can help to prevent night blindness. Although spinach
provides an exceptional source of calcium, it is also high in
oxalic acid, which can partly interfere with the absorption
of the calcium.

Caution: People with a tendency to kidney stones
should eat spinach sparingly, since its high oxalic acid can
tend to form calcium-oxalate kidney stones in susceptible
individuals.

SPIRULINA

Spirulina is a blue-green, single-cell algae, which is spiral-
shaped – hence its name. It thrives in warm alkaline lakes
such as Lake Chad in Africa and Lake Texcoco in Mexico.
The algae, which appears to be a floating green scum, is
collected from the lake and dried. Spirulina was so highly
valued as a sustaining food by the ancient Aztecs, that it was
used by them as currency – and modern science has recently
discovered why. Spirulina contains over 65 per cent complete
protein, a rarity among plant foods, and this protein, which
is predigested by the algae, is so well-balanced that it is easier
to digest than meat. Spirulina absorbs and retains many minerals from the lakes, including potassium, calcium, zinc,

magnesium, manganese, selenium, iron and phosphorus. In addition, it is a rich source of the B vitamins, including usable amounts of B12, as well as vitamin E, beta carotene, GLA (essential fatty acid) and chlorophyll.

Spirulina has tonifying and cleansing properties and can be used to detoxify the liver and kidneys, cleanse the arteries, build and enrich the blood and promote intestinal flora. It is also very beneficial for weight control, not only because it is a low-calorie nutrient, but also because it contains high amounts of phenylalanine, the amino acid which curbs the appetite.

Spirulina has been used in the treatment of anaemia, weakness, malnutrition, hepatitis, inner inflammations, diabetes, hypoglycaemia and poor skin tone. It is a versatile food supplement which strengthens the immune system and increases resistance to disease and inflammations. It also contains a blue pigment, phycocyanin, which is a protein known to inhibit cancer. Since it is grown and harvested in unpolluted areas, totally free of environmental pollutants, spirulina is one of the safest foods available. It is sold in health food shops in both powder and tablet form.

SPROUTS

Sprouts (young shoots from recently germinated seeds), mainly **soybean**, have been a part of the Chinese diet for thousands of years. Sprouts are rich in chlorophyll, vitamins A, C, D, E, K and B complex, and in minerals such as calcium, phosphorus, potassium, magnesium and iron. They are also abundant in quality protein and enzymes, making them easily digestible. Sprouts have been described as 'the most living food in the world' since, unlike most plants, they are eaten at the peak of their freshness and vitality while they are still growing, and anyone who eats sprouts regularly will experience this vitality and increased energy. Sprouts are diuretics, appetizers and detoxify the body. They are used for weight loss, arthritis, oedema, peptic and duodenal ulcers, and by people with weak digestion.

Miraculous things happen when grain or legume seeds begin to germinate – the starches and oils contained in the seeds are converted to vitamins, proteins, enzymes and simple sugars. For example, vitamin C increases six-fold so that a 100 g serving of soybean sprouts will contain 120 mg vitamin C, which is double the recommended daily amount. The protein content of alfalfa sprouts rises to between 16 and 31 per cent, and their carotene content equals that of carrots. The B vitamins, enzymes and other nutrients also increase spectacularly, making sprouts an easily digested form of nourishment.

Alfalfa sprouts are among the most popular and, because they contain more minerals, they are more nutritious than other sprouts. The roots of the alfalfa plant can penetrate as deeply as 100 feet, where access to minerals is highest, and thus the sprout can contain concentrated amounts of iron, calcium, magnesium, potassium, zinc, phosphorus, sodium, sulphur, silicon, chlorine and cobalt.

Sprouts are commonly sold in both health food shops and supermarkets. Seeds such as peas, chickpeas, wheat sesame and corn are easily sprouted at home using plastic sprouters available in health food stores.

SQUASH, WINTER

A gourd-shaped vegetable native to North America, winter

squashes provide an outstanding source of alpha and beta carotenes (provitamin A), and contain good amounts of calcium, phosphorus and potassium. Squashes can benefit the stomach, reduce inflammations and improve circulation and squash seeds are reputed to be effective in destroying worms. Some healers recommend that, a handful of seeds should be eaten daily for three weeks in order to eliminate parasitic worms.

ST JOHN'S WORT *(HYPERICUM PERFORATUM)*

A yellow-flowered herb, which is both cultivated and found wild in the UK and Europe, infusions of the flowers can have a beneficial effect on metabolism and bile secretion. They also improve circulation, have a general anti-inflammatory effect, stimulate appetite, relieve depression and promote sleep. Infusions can also be used externally to bathe wounds, haemorrhoids and burns. A tea of the leaves is said to stimulate expulsion of phlegm or mucus, and is beneficial in coughs. Available from health food stores and in nutritional formulas.

STINGING NETTLE SEE NETTLE

SUGAR SEE CARBOHYDRATES

SULPHUR

Dubbed as 'the beauty mineral', sulphur is important for smooth, glossy hair, as well as for healthy skin and nails. It is a non-metallic mineral, abundant in nature and present in every cell. It is needed for the formation of collagen, one of the most prevalent proteins, which is found in skin, bone and cartilage. As such, sulphur contributes to a healthy look-ing skin. It also has a laxative effect due to its ability to absorb water in the intestines – Epsom salts are in fact sul-phates of magnesium.

Sulphur detoxifies the body, cleans the arteries and helps the body to rid itself of damaging toxic elements. Together with proteins, sulphur forms the vitally important 'sulphur-containing amino acids', cysteine, taurine and methionine. Cysteine and methionine are needed to form the important anti-ageing, antioxidant enzymes which neutralize danger-ous peroxide free radicals and help to prevent the degenera-tive diseases of ageing, such as arthritis. In fact, sulphur has long been known to benefit arthritis, and one of its best sources is eggs, which are high in sulphur-containing cys-teine. Used externally, in ointments and in the spa waters of regions such as the Dead Sea, sulphur has traditionally been considered beneficial for the treatment of psoriasis, eczema and dermatitis.

Deficiency symptoms of sulphur can include arthritis, dry hair, brittle nails and rough skin. Some of the best nat-ural sources of the mineral are eggs, meat, onions, alfalfa, broccoli, cabbage and watercress.

SUNFLOWER SEED and OIL

Sunflowers, which originated in North America and were cultivated by the American Indians, were first introduced into Europe in the sixteenth century. Nowadays, vast fields of the brilliant golden flowers are a familiar sight across many European landscapes in the summer months.

Sunflower seeds are sun-energized nutritional power-houses and it is no wonder that in pre-revolutionary Russia field soldiers received a kilo of sunflower seeds as emergency rations on which to subsist if stranded. The seeds are rich in protein (24 per cent), polyunsaturated fatty acids (66 per cent), vitamins A, E, D and several B vitamins, calcium, magnesium, phosphorus, iron, zinc, potassium, fluorine and iodine.

Sunflower seeds can be used as a snack, a topping for salads, as a nut butter spread, or included in bread. The seeds have been described as beneficial to eyesight, skin and fingernails and useful adjuncts in the treatment of hypertension and irritated nerves. Sprouted sunflower seeds are easily digestible and rich in vitamin E, lecithin and pectin. As a supplement, two tablespoonfuls of sunflower seeds a day are recommended, even for people on reducing diets. Both are widely available.

Sunflower seed oil is one of the richest sources of essential fatty acids. It contains as much as 66 per cent essential polyunsaturated fatty acids, and has the highest content of all seeds of the essential linoleic acid. The oil can be used as an all-purpose kitchen oil, although it is best used fresh and raw as a base in salad dressings to obtain its full nutritional value. It can also be blended with butter, thereby enriching the butter with its essential fatty acids.

SWEET POTATOES AND YAMS

A vegetable with large, fleshy, edible roots, sweet potatoes are believed to have originated in South America. Today, they are grown throughout the world and are an important food in many countries – about 85 per cent of the world's sweet potato crop is grown in China.

Outstandingly rich in vitamin A (many times more so than potatoes), sweet potatoes also provide vitamin C, calcium, iron, potassium, phosphorus and sodium, but they must be baked or boiled in their skins to retain these nutrients. Due to their exceptional content of vitamin A, sweet potatoes can be used to improve night vision. They are also reported to increase milk secretion in nursing mothers, remove toxins from the body and treat underweight and diarrhoea.

Sweet potatoes are best selected when fresh looking, firm to the touch, and preferably either with a dark grey skin colour (yams) or red skin colour (sweet potatoes) – most 'yams' sold in the US are in fact sweet potatoes with red flesh. The vegetables should not be refrigerated as this can cause chilling injuries. However, if stored in a cool dry place, they can be kept for several months. They are widely available.

Caution: Since sweet potatoes can cause indigestion and abdominal swelling, they should be eaten in moderate servings.

T

TAHINI SEE SESAME

TAMARIND *(TAMARINDUS INDICA)*

An evergreen tree native to India, it bears small, sweet fruits in pods. Tamarind fruit is well known as a gentle laxative and is sometimes used as an ingredient in laxative preparations. The leaves are reputed to destroy parasitic intestinal worms. In Asia, tamarind fruit is eaten as a food; it is also made into a refreshing and cooling beverage, which is particularly suitable for people with fever. Tamarind is exported and available in specialist shops in the West.

TARRAGON *(ARTEMISIA DRACUNCULUS)*

A green perennial shrub, its aromatic leaves are commonly used as a culinary herb. The fresh leaves and oil are used in tarragon mustard and tarragon vinegar, and also in the cooking of fish or chicken. Infusions of tarragon leaves can be used to stimulate digestive secretions and appetite, relieve digestive disorders, bring on delayed menstruation, and promote urination by stimulating the kidneys. Tarragon tea, taken at bedtime, can help to relieve insomnia.

TAURINE

Taurine is a sulphur-containing, non-essential amino acid. However, it is one of the most abundant **amino acids** in the body and an **antioxidant** which neutralizes free radicals. It also helps to raise **calcium** levels in the body by transporting calcium (and sodium) across the intestinal wall into the bloodstream. In addition, taurine is a component of **bile**, which is essential for the digestion of fats, absorption of fat-soluble vitamins and controlling cholesterol levels. Taurine is produced in the body from cysteine with the help of vitamin B6, and is concentrated in excitable tissues such as the heart, muscles and nerve tissues, but it is not commonly found in food. It is thought to have an inhibitory action on epilepsy and has been used to reduce seizures. Its inhibitory action can also help to counteract anxiety and stress, especially when combined with histidine and glycine. Taurine is available as a food supplement and beneficial levels range between 500 and 3,000 mg daily.

TEA *(CAMELLIA SINENSIS)*

The tea plant is an evergreen that is grown in many tropical and subtropical regions of the world, particularly in India and China, which together produce the bulk of the world's tea supplies. The flavours of the teas produced vary from country to country, and are dependent not only on soil type and processing methods, but also on the elevation of the plantations, with the finest tea coming from higher, cooler areas, as the plant grows more slowly in cool air, adding to its flavour.

Black tea is a stimulating, refreshing and diuretic beverage provided it is not strongly steeped, only lightly infused.

It is traditionally used to aid digestion, especially after a heavy meal; it also relieves thirst, removes flatulence and counteracts diarrhoea. A popular tea variety, 'Earl Grey', consists of black tea blended with bergamot oil, which is in itself refreshing, relaxing and calming, and adds these properties in the blending to the tea.

Common tea contains stimulating and astringent substances, including theophylline, theine and tannins, which are known to stimulate overproduction of cellular products, such as fibrous tissue and cyst fluid. Strong tea is medicinally used to halt dysentery and treat chronic inflammations such as gastritis and enteritis. It is also used externally for certain skin conditions.

Excessive drinking of tea has been found to contribute to constipation, nervousness, breast lumps and, in sensitive individuals, to mimic the many symptoms of irritable bowel syndrome.

Some milder types of tea, which are made from the branches of certain tea plants, are exported from Japan and marketed as 'bancha twig tea' or 'kukicha'. (See also GREEN TEA)

TEA TREE OIL (MELALEUCA ALTERNEFOLIA)

Tea tree is a native of Australia where it is cultivated especially for its valuable oil, which is extracted from the leaves by steam distillation. This oil has been found to be an effective antiseptic, with strong germicidal and fungicidal actions.

For many years, the Australian aboriginals bathed in the healing waters of swampy areas in which the tea tree grew. They used the plant on their skins by crushing the leaves and spreading the pulp on affected areas. When discovered in 1700 by British explorers, tea tree was named by Captain Cook when he observed the aboriginals brewing tea from the leaves. Since then, the tea tree has been studied scientifically and found to contain 48 compounds, including terpine 4-ol, one of its most therapeutic ingredients. These compounds, not all of which have been identified, have been found to be beneficial in healing infected wounds, skin inflammations, carbuncles and pus-filled infections; as such, they were used during World War II by Australian troops. Tea tree oil has since been found to be very beneficial in the treatment of various conditions such as bladder inflammation (cystitis), athlete's foot, diaper rash, insect bites, sunburns, cuts, fungi, dandruff and itchy scalp.

Nowadays, tea tree oil is incorporated into many personal care products, such as dandruff shampoos and conditioners, deodorants, toothpastes, antiseptic mouthwashes, ointments for treating acne and fungal infections, and as a douche for vaginal yeast infections.

TEMPEH

The most popular soya food in Indonesia, tempeh originated in Java more than 200 years ago and is now sold in thousands of shops in Java alone, and in increasing numbers of health food shops in the US and other Western countries.

Tempeh is a fermented soya product made from cooked soybeans bound together by a dense fungus (rhizopus) and then moulded into compact patties. Sold fresh, refrigerated or frozen, the patties can be sliced and fried until crisp, and their flavour and texture resemble southern fried chicken. Different varieties of tempeh are produced by combining the soybeans with grains such as wheat, rice, millet or coconut.

Soya tempeh is highly nutritious. It contains 18 per cent protein and is an exceptional vegetarian source of vitamin B12. Popular Western recipes include Tempeh Burgers, Seasoned Crisp Tempeh and Tempeh Sandwiches.

THEOBROMINE

An ingredient found mainly in cocoa and chocolate, theobromine is a stimulating alkaloid and one of the methylxanthines, a group of compounds which include caffeine and theophylline. Theobromine expands blood vessels in the heart, increases urination, reduces calcium absorption, and is a mild stimulator of the nervous system. It is known to stimulate overproduction of cellular products, such as fibrous tissue and cyst fluid.

THEOPHYLLINE

An alkaloid found in **tea**, theophylline is a methylxanthine, diuretic and a mild stimulator.

THIAMINE SEE VITAMIN B1

THREONINE

An essential amino acid which helps to maintain protein balance in the body, it is important for the synthesis of collagen.

Threonine is concentrated in the heart, nervous system and skeletal muscles and also helps the liver to handle fats in combination with **aspartic acid** and **methionine**.

THYME *(THYMUS VULGARIS)*

A small, scented garden plant which is native to the Mediterranean regions, thyme was used by the Romans, both as a culinary and therapeutic herb. Its aromatic and spicy tasting leaves, which are rich in essential oils, are used in cooking and in infusions. Thyme is a good tonic for the stomach and nerves. Its tea relieves flatulence, promotes appetite, strengthens digestion, loosens phlegm and increases perspiration. Infusions have a calming effect, relax muscle spasms and alleviate exhaustion. Extracts and infusions are also used to treat bronchitis, laryngitis and coughs. Thyme vinegar was used for centuries to relieve headaches. Essential oil of thyme makes a good antiseptic mouthwash, and is also used externally for warts and for a relaxing bath.

Caution: Too much thyme can overstimulate the thyroid and cause poisoning symptoms.

TOCOPHEROL SEE VITAMIN E

TOFU

A common staple of Japanese cuisine, tofu is a cheese-like soybean curd which has now become extremely popular in West countries and various types, such as silken tofu, firm tofu or tofu puddings, are currently available in health food shops.

Tofu has been praised for its high protein content of 35 per cent, and for its high protein quality, which includes all the essential amino acids. Indeed, many people in Asia depend on tofu for their daily protein, and it is now considered to be an ideal replacement for meat, thus allowing more people to become vegetarians. As a serving of 8 ounces provides only 147 calories, it is ideal as a diet food – an equal amount of beef would contain five times as many calories. Tofu is also low in saturated fats and cholesterol, it is rich in calcium, and it is a good source of the B vitamins, vitamin E, potassium and sodium. As such, it is beneficial for conditions such as diabetes, heart disease and atherosclerosis.

Fresh tofu will keep for about five to seven days when refrigerated, deep-fried tofu will keep up to ten days, while special types of silken tofu can be kept sealed in their containers for up to six months. Available from health food stores and supermarkets.

TOMATOES

Tomatoes originated in South America and were brought to Europe from Mexico in the mid-sixteenth century. They are rich in vitamins A and C and a good source of calcium, phosphorus, potassium and sodium. They detoxify the body, purify the blood, strengthen digestion and are useful in cases of poor appetite, poor digestion or constipation. Although tomatoes are considered an acidic food, they alkalize the blood after digestion and are useful in treating acidic conditions such as gout. Tomatoes contain lycopene, a powerful antioxidant which neutralizes damaging free radicals. Lycopene has been found to be outstandingly effective in quenching singlet oxygen, which is a very reactive type of free radical that damages the **DNA** blueprint (which supervises cell division), causing mutations and cancer. In fact, the results of one study have indicated that increasing dietary lycopene levels may provide a significant protector from digestive tract cancers. Lycopene is now being incorporated as an ingredient in various multivitamin preparations.

Caution: Tomatoes can interfere with calcium absorption and should be avoided in cases of arthritis. More than four tomatoes a day are not recommended.

TRYPSIN

A protein–splitting enzyme secreted by the pancreas, trypsin enables the digestion of proteins in the intestines. It is included in many digestive-aid tablets such as **pancreatin**.

TRYPTOPHAN

An essential amino acid, tryptophan has several crucial roles. It is used to form structural protein in the body, manufacture antibodies, produce vitamin B3 (niacin), and create serotonin, which is an inhibitory neurotransmitter – a brain chemical that conveys calming messages between brain cells. Serotonin induces sleep at night and relaxation during the day. It helps to alleviate stress, control hyperactivity in children, stabilize blood pressure, protect the heart and aids weight control. Tryptophan needs vitamin B6 and C to be converted to serotonin, and adequate level of vitamin B3 is also important. When these are in short supply, less serotonin is available, and this is manifested by symptoms such as insomnia, depression, anxiety and hypertension.

Tryptophan is no longer available as food supplement. It

was banned in 1989 because a few contaminated batches, produced in Japan by genetic engineering, caused the outbreak of a rare disease (EMS), resulting in the death of 24 people. Although tryptophan itself was not to blame, only the new manufacturing process, sales of tryptophan are still banned. Tryptophan is plentiful in foods such as milk, turkey and bananas, while a glass of milk at bedtime is known to help induce sleep.

TURMERIC (CURCUMA LONGA)

A common culinary spice, its source is the roots of a plant which is native to Asia. Turmeric was traditionally used by both Indian and Chinese systems of medicine to treat inflammations and cure sprains. It contains a yellow pigment, curcumin, which is an active ingredient that has been used for centuries, not only to season foods, but also as a food preservative and colouring agent. The curcuminoids in turmeric are a group of phenolic acids which have been found to have unique antioxidant and anti-inflammatory properties. They retard age-related diseases by preventing free radical damage, inhibit the growth of cancer cells, protect the liver from toxins, help to dissolve gallstones, lower cholesterol levels, alleviate joint swellings, increase joint flexibility and reduce menstrual pain. Studies with HIV patients have shown that turmeric also has a beneficial effect in the treatment of AIDS.

Used externally in a poultice, turmeric mixed with lime is an ancient household remedy for sprains, muscular pain and inflamed joints. It is available as a nutritional supplement in capsule form.

TURNIPS

A member of the mustard family, the turnip is a root vegetable which is rich in vitamins A and C, and minerals such
as sulphur, calcium, potassium, sodium and phosphorus.
Turnips detoxify the body and alkalize the blood, promote
sweating, releasing mucus and improving the appetite. They
are also generally beneficial in conditions such as indigestion, diabetes and jaundice. Turnips have traditionally been
used in Asia in the treatment of lung congestions, bronchitis,
asthma and sinus problems. Although raw turnips have a
somewhat pungent smell, this is destroyed in cooking.

TYROSINE, L-TYROSINE

A non-essential amino acid, tyrosine has many vital effects
in the body such as fighting depression, maintaining energy
and controlling weight. Together with iodine, tyrosine produces thyroxine, the vital thyroid hormone which controls
the rate of metabolism, weight, energy and growth. With
phenylalanine, tyrosine produces norepinephrine (adrenalin)
and dopamine, two important neurotransmitters – the
chemicals which enable brain cells to communicate with
each other. Norepinephrine is important in the control of
stress, anxiety, fatigue and allergies, while dopamine controls
motivation, movement and emotions. Tyrosine participates
in the production of endorphins, the brain's natural pain
relievers and mood elevators. Tyrosine is abundant in animal
food and is also available as a nutritional supplement from
health food stores.

Caution: Tyrosine should not be used by people with
melanoma.

U/V

UVA URSI SEE BEARBERRY

VALERIAN *(VALERIANA OFFICINALIS)*

A wild herb with fragrant flowers, valerian is cultivated for its root and its essential oil. A tincture of the oil is well known as a strong sedative that counteracts anxiety, calms nervousness, reduces heart palpitations, spasms and epileptic fits. Valerian is a wonderfully soothing herb which promotes sleep and is a good painkiller. Traditionally used to prevent fainting, valerian can help in the treatment of digestive ulcers and reduce the urge to smoke. Available from health food stores, pharmacies and herbalists. Also widely incorporated in nutritional formulas.

Caution: Valerian should not be prepared as a tea unless prescribed by a doctor. Prolonged use of the herb can cause depression.

VALINE

An essential amino acid needed for the formation of protein in the body, valine has a stimulating effect. It is one of the three branched chain amino acids and, in combination with the other two, **leucine** and isoleucine, valine benefits muscles. It assists the repair of muscle tissue in cases of injuries. Available from health food stores and in nutritional formulas.

VANADIUM

Vanadium has recently been discovered as an essential nutrient in human nutrition. Named after the Scandinavian goddess of beauty, vanadium is a trace element which appears to improve insulin action. Vanadium supplements (mostly as vanadyl sulphate) have improved glucose tolerance in animals, inhibited cholesterol and increased bone mineralization. As a result, vanadyl sulphate is now commonly used by diabetics. Vanadyl sulphate is found in many foods. Its best sources include buckwheat, parsley, mushrooms, black pepper, dill and shellfish. No deficiency symptoms have been noted so far and as yet no recommended daily allowance for the nutrient has been set, but an intake of between 10 and 60 mcg a day is considered normal.

VEGAN DIET

The vegan diet is a strict form of vegetarianism which promotes the use of fruits, vegetables and spring water, and excludes any animal foods, even those accepted by many vegetarians, such as dairy foods or eggs.

Vegan diets have proved beneficial in detoxifying the blood, preventing various diseases such as hypertension, high cholesterol, heart disease, cancer and osteoporosis and curing inflammations and allergic conditions such as asthma and hay fever. Allergies and inflammations are known to arise from leukotrienes, metabolic derivatives of arachidonic acid. This is an essential fatty acid found exclusively in animal products. The elimination of animal products, as in the vegan diet, is thought to prevent the formation of leukotrienes and their related diseases. Obviously, a strict, long-term vegan diet is not suitable for everyone, and could create deficiencies in nutrients such as **vitamin B12**, **zinc** and **proteins**, leading to fatigue and anaemia. However, this effect can be avoided by the use of concentrated foods such as **brewer's yeast**, **bee pollen**, **spirulina**, **blue–green algae**, **chlorella**, or by taking supplements. Another way to avoid protein deficiency among vegans is to eat the correct plant protein combinations, for instance, by combining grains and legumes at the same meal and in the correct proportions to yield usable protein (see *Complete Nutrition*). Soya products such as **miso** and **tofu** are also very helpful for increasing protein intake. It should be remembered, however, that nutrient requirements vary from person to person, and that for many people strict dietary restrictions can cause nutrient shortages and deficiency symptoms unless supplements are used.

VEGETARIAN DIET

A vegetarian diet excludes the use of animal meats, but not necessarily the use of other animal foods such as eggs, **milk**, **yogurt** and **cheese**. It depends on the individual interpretation of vegetarianism. However, all vegetarian diets are high in fibre and, usually, the protein problem is less acute than in the vegan diet, since vegetarians use some animal protein, which supplies vitamin B12, and they also use high–protein soya products freely, such as **tofu** and **miso**. In general, vegetarian diets have been shown to be effective in lowering high cholesterol levels and hypertension, preventing atherosclerosis and heart disease, alleviating constipation, reducing the risk of colon cancer, breast cancer and kidney stones. A vegetarian diet can also help to prevent osteoporosis, since a high protein diet and sugar are known to increase excretion of calcium in the urine.

VERVAIN, VERBENA *(VERBENA OFFICINALIS)*

A herb which grows wild in meadows and roadside verges, it is also widely cultivated as a garden plant. It was traditionally regarded as a 'sacred' herb, and infusions of verbena leaves are used by both herbalists and homeopaths. Taken in a single dose, these infusions are diuretic; they loosen phlegm so that it can be coughed up, stimulate vomiting, promote perspiration, relieve indigestion, and can benefit ulcers and colitis. Vervain is also a sedative, relieving depression and anxiety, inducing sleep and alleviating certain types of migraines.

VINE LEAVES *(VITIS VINIFERA)*

Vine leaves are commonly used in Mediterranean cooking and contain important **bioflavonoids**, such as anthocyanidins which are potent **antioxidants**, and other flavonoids. These factors promote blood circulation, strengthen veins and capillaries and help retain their flexibility. The leaves are also recommended in the treatment of varicose veins and haemorrhoids. Available from specialist ethnic grocers.

VITAMIN A

Vitamin A is an **antioxidant**, fat-soluble vitamin which occurs in two forms. In animal foods such as fish oils and liver, it occurs as **retinol** which is readily used by the body, or stored in the liver. In vegetable foods, it occurs as **beta carotene** and other **carotenoids** (provitamin A) which must first be converted in the body to retinol, before becoming usable as vitamin A.

Vitamin A is important for growth, development and fertility. It boosts the immune system and helps to fight colds, increasing resistance to infections of mucous tissue linings such as eyes, ears, throat, lungs and bladder. Together with beta carotene it improves vision, especially night vision, by forming a photosensitive pigment called visual purple. Vitamin A maintains a healthy-looking skin, preventing acne, dermatitis and skin cancer. High doses of retinol and beta carotene can also prevent cancer of lungs, bladder and breasts. Deficiency symptoms include red itchy eyes, impaired vision, dry or rough skin and a predisposition to colds and infections.

Vitamin A is stored in the liver until needed and, in spite of its wide prevalence, deficiencies do occur. Most vulnerable are dieters, people on low fat regimes or vegans, since only a small part of the beta carotene is converted to retinol if the fat intake is low. Vitamin A supplements are therefore important in unbalanced diets. The recommended daily allowance for adults is 5,000 i.u., and for children 3,000 i.u. Requirements increase during illness, but decrease when using oral contraceptives. Most nutritionists recommend a daily dose of 10,000 i.u. for adults. Excessive doses of the order of 50,000 i.u., taken regularly over periods of a few months, can produce toxic effects.

VITAMIN B COMPLEX

B complex is a group of water-soluble B vitamins which occur together in many vegetables and animal foods. Rich sources include liver, brewer's yeast, raw wheat germ and brown rice. Although certain functions of many B vitamins overlap, all have their own characteristics and they cannot replace one another. Moreover, they interact with each other in many bodily functions. They are vital for such activities as energy production, carbohydrate metabolism and proper nerve function. They have a wide range of effects, from alleviating stress to preventing atherosclerosis. Their deficiency symptoms include fatigue, nervousness, depression, anaemia, weak digestion, poor appetite, constipation, hair loss and high cholesterol levels.

B vitamins are depleted by refined sugar and flour, and by alcohol and, being water-soluble, the B vitamins in raw vegetables readily dissolve into the cooking water, enriching the soup or cooking liquid. It is important therefore to save the cooking water of vegetables or brown rice as this provides a rich source of B vitamins. When taking supplements of B vitamins, it is best to consume the whole B complex. Excessive supplementation of only one of the B vitamins disrupts the balance and can promote elimination of the others. When a specific B vitamin is needed to treat a particular condition, say B6 for dieting, it is best to take an additional source of B complex in order to maintain a proper balance of the other B vitamins.

VITAMIN B1 *(THIAMINE)*

This was the first B vitamin to be identified and, as it was discovered in rice husks, thiamine became commonly known as the cure for beri-beri, a fatal Asian disease caused by eating polished rice. It was realized that the symptoms of beri-beri, such as mental disturbances, muscle wasting, hypertension and heart attacks, could be cured simply by eating raw brown rice.

As a **coenzyme**, thiamine is essential for energy production, carbohydrate metabolism and nerve function. As an **antioxidant**, it can help to prevent arthritis and atherosclerosis caused by free radical damage. Together with **vitamin C** and cysteine, thiamine also helps to protect from the damage caused by smoking and smog.

Thiamine has been called the 'morale vitamin' due to its salutary effect on the nerves. It promotes a feeling of optimism, helps to overcome stress, depression, anxiety and poor memory, stabilizes appetite and maintains normal heart function; it is important to growth, lactation and fertility. Deficiency symptoms include fatigue, water retention, poor appetite, heart palpitations, low thyroid function, nervous exhaustion, irritability, fear, anxiety and confusion. Among the best natural sources of thiamine are brewer's yeast, rice bran, raw wheat germ, whole grains, peanuts and green and yellow vegetables. The vitamin is destroyed by alcohol, coffee, tea and raw uncooked fish.

The recommended daily allowance is 1.4 mg for adults and 0.7 mg for children, but many people use supplements containing 50 mg to ensure a feeling of well-being. Requirements increase during stress, lactation or illness.

VITAMIN B2 *(RIBOFLAVIN)*

First identified as the yellow-green pigment in milk, riboflavin is vital for metabolism and energy production. Together with vitamin A, it contributes to good vision and promotes growth and fertility. Large doses have been reported to prevent athlete's foot, improve eczemas and allergies and counteract a sweet tooth.

Riboflavin is not destroyed by cooking, but it is sensitive to light – which is why milk, which is a good source of riboflavin, should not be kept in clear containers or exposed to strong sunlight.

Riboflavin deficiency symptoms include the cracking of the lips at the corner of the mouth, tongue inflammations, a sensation of sand in the eyes, cataracts, migraine, scaly skin on the face, dental problems, anaemia and heart disease. Among the best natural sources of the vitamin are milk, liver, brewer's yeast, dairy products, green leafy vegetables, fish and eggs. The recommended daily allowance is 1.7 mg for adults and 1 mg for children, although most popular supplements contain 50 mg. Since riboflavin is excreted through the kidneys, excessive consumption or supplementation will result in yellowish-green urine, but this is perfectly normal.

VITAMIN B3 *(NIACIN)*

Also called nicotinic acid, niacin was discovered whilst searching for the cause of pellagra, a common endemic disease of the eighteenth century, which is characterized by the three Ds – dermatitis, dementia and diarrhoea. It is a water-soluble vitamin available in two forms, niacin and niacinamide.

Niacin assists metabolism, digestion and energy production and improves blood circulation, preventing blood clots and heart attacks; it lowers high cholesterol levels safely and effectively when taken in daily doses of 3 g or more and is vital to a healthy nervous system, alleviating nervousness, mental disorders and suicidal tendencies. It also enhances insulin secretion and has been reported to benefit new cases of diabetes. In higher doses of 50 mg, niacin releases histamine which produces a temporary hot skin flush for a few minutes. This reaction can be prevented by using niacinamide instead of niacin or by using 'flush free' niacin products. (Histamine is a chemical released during allergic reactions, but which is also vital to various functions of the body such as growth, wound healing and orgasm).

Severe deficiencies of niacin can bring about the symptoms of pellagra, although nowadays this is somewhat rare. However, lower deficiencies are very common and symptoms can include fatigue, indigestion, bad breath, arthritis, headaches, high cholesterol levels, headaches and lost sense of humour.

Megadoses of a few grams of niacin a day have been used successfully to treat mental cases of depression and schizophrenia and it is assumed that such illnesses are indicative of a much higher requirement for niacin. Niacin supplements have also been used to treat alcoholism and smoking.

Among the best natural sources of niacin are liver, brewer's yeast, eggs, fish, rice bran, wheat bran, peanuts, sunflower seeds and wheat germ. The recommended daily allowance is 20 mg for adults and 13 mg for children. However, niacin supplementation of between 50 and 100 mg a day can be safely used for greater benefits. Niacin and niacinamide supplements are available on their own or included in B complex or multivitamin formulations. Niacin supplements are best taken with meals.

VITAMIN B5 SEE PANTOTHENIC ACID

VITAMIN B6 *(PYRIDOXINE)*

One of the busiest of the B vitamins, pyridoxine is an **antioxidant** vitamin and is involved with more than sixty **enzymes**, taking part in many and varied metabolic functions. It promotes muscle energy by releasing stored sugar from the liver; it helps to metabolize fats and control obesity, lowers cholesterol and prevents atherosclerosis; it regulates the sodium–potassium balance, preventing water-retention; it maintains a correct acid–alkaline ratio and assists the functions of nerves. Pyridoxine also inhibits the release of histamine and is therefore beneficial to asthmatics and allergy sufferers, and it helps to synthesize nucleic acids, antibodies and red blood cells. In addition, it promotes healthy pregnancies, strengthens the immune system and assists blood formation. Pyridoxine supplements of 50 mg daily can effectively prevent morning sickness in pregnancy, and higher doses of 200 mg daily are reported to be effective in treating the carpal tunnel syndrome, reducing the need for surgeries. Pyridoxine is also involved in brain chemistry, promoting the production of neurotransmitters such as serotonin, and it has been found helpful for controlling occurrences of epileptic seizures. Together with magnesium, pyridoxine inhibits the formation of oxalic acid salts, such as calcium oxalate, thus helping to prevent kidney stones.

Pyridoxine is not stored in the body, and is depleted in milk by pasteurization, partially destroyed by cooking, and mostly removed from grains by refining. Alcohol and oral contraceptive pills are among its greatest antagonists, and any woman on the pill should consider taking pyridoxine-supplements. Deficiency symptoms include water retention, linear nail ridges, tongue inflammations, inability to tan, numbness of hands and feet, convulsions in children, depression, tremors, hypoglycaemia, diabetes, appetite loss, high cholesterol levels, kidney stones, osteoporosis, arthritis, allergies, asthma, anaemia and poor dream recollection.

Some of the best natural sources of pyrodoxine are brewer's yeast, liver and kidney, sunflower seeds, raw wheat germ, walnuts, molasses, cabbage, milk and eggs. The recommended daily allowance for adults is 2.2 mg, and 1.7 mg for children. The normal nutritional supplementation range is between 50 and 100 mg daily. As it is a water-soluble vitamin, pyridoxine supplementation is best divided throughout the day and taken at intervals.

VITAMIN B12 (COBALAMIN)

Isolated from liver extract in 1948, vitamin B12 was identified as the food factor that prevents the fatal condition pernicious anaemia. The vitamin is water soluble and contains the mineral cobalt, hence its name. It comes in several forms, of which cyanocobalamin is the most common.

Although cobalamin is required in tiny amounts, measured in micrograms, it is essential for the functioning of all cells and is principally involved in energy metabolism, immune function and nerve function. Together with folic acid, the vitamin forms red blood cells to prevent anaemia, and promotes growth and appetite in children, increases energy, improves brain functions such as memory and learning ability, maintains a healthy nervous system, stabilizes menstruation and prevents post-natal depression. Vitamin B12 is used to treat a wide range of conditions, such as fatigue, depression, Alzheimer's disease, asthma, infertility, multiple sclerosis, noise-induced hearing loss and AIDS.

The absorption of B12 depends on a stomach secretion called the 'intrinsic factor'. Many people with reduced secretion suffer unknowingly from a deficiency of the vitamin, which can take years to manifest, since B12 is stored in the liver – unlike the other water-soluble vitamins. B12 deficiency is thought to be especially common in the elderly, and affects primarily the brain and nervous system. Apart from fatigue and depression, deficiency symptoms include a pins-and-needles sensation, impaired memory, red tongue, diarrhoea, shortness of breath, heart palpitation and apathy. More acute deficiencies include symptoms such as loss of co-ordination and senile dementia.

B12 is only found in significant quantities in animal foods, and its richest sources are liver, kidneys, sardines, eggs, fish and cheese. In non-animal foods, B12 is found in fermented soya products (**miso, tofu, tempeh**), algae (**spirulina, chlorella, blue-green algae**) and **bee pollen**. **Vegans** and strict **vegetarians** are well-advised to take B12 supplements to prevent deficiencies. The recommended daily allowance is 2 mcg for adults and 1 mcg for children. Supplements are available in potencies of between 60 mcg and 2,000 mcg. Some people are not able to absorb B12 easily, and therefore need to take high supplementary dosages, either orally or by injection.

VITAMIN B15 SEE PANGAMIC ACID

VITAMIN C *(ASCORBIC ACID)*

Vitamin C is a water-soluble nutrient which was first recognized as a cure for scurvy, long before it was isolated in 1933. In recent years, it has received a great deal of public attention as a cure for the common cold. But vitamin C does much more than just prevent scurvy or colds. For example, as an **antioxidant**, it delays ageing and prevents age-related diseases, from arthritis to Parkinson's disease; as an antihistamine, it alleviates allergies; and as an antipollutant, it eliminates toxins from the body.

However, the chief function of vitamin C is the production of collagen, the structural protein which holds our bodies together. As such, it hastens the healing of wounds, prevents bleeding gums and strengthens capillaries and blood vessels, preventing heart attacks and strokes. Collagen is also the subcutaneous 'cement', and facial wrinkles can be a sign of a life-long deficiency in vitamin C. Vitamin C is also a powerful booster of the immune system and is well known for its ability to increase resistance to infections and disease by increasing the production of antibodies and interferon, which fight microbes and viruses. Scientific studies have confirmed that megadoses of vitamin C can reduce the risk of a wide range of cancers, and also inhibit tumour development and prolong the survival of cancer patients. In dosages of at least 1,000 mg a day, vitamin C helps to lower cholesterol by speeding its conversion to bile. Vitamin C also aids the absorption of iron, preventing anaemia and provides protection against the devastating effects of smoking and alcoholism.

Deficiency symptoms of vitamin C include susceptibility to colds, infections and allergies, easy bruising and the slow healing of wounds, inflamed gums and defective teeth, fatigue and anaemia, and nervousness, anxiety and depression. Among the best natural sources of the vitamin are fresh citrus fruits, peppers, guavas, broccoli, Brussels sprouts, cabbage, papaya and kiwi. The natural vitamin C in fruits and vegetables is highly perishable as the vitamin is unstable and disintegrates, not only in cooking, but also in peeled fruits and vegetables.

The recommended daily allowances of vitamin C are 60 mg for adults and 45 mg for children. However, these are ridiculously low dosages that can mainly prevent scurvy. For optimal benefits, doses of a few grams a day are recommended. Vitamin C tablets which contain **bioflavonoids** are preferable.

VITAMIN D

Vitamin D is a fat soluble vitamin, supplied either by food or exposure to the sun. It is known as the 'sunshine vitamin' since the sun's ultra violet rays convert subcutaneous cholesterol to vitamin D. There are two major forms of vitamin D – D2 (ergocalciferol) and D3 (cholecalciferol); vitamin D2 is the form added to milk and used in nutritional supplements.

Vitamin D promotes absorption of calcium and phosphorus, both of which are vital for strong bones and teeth and for preventing rickets in children. Vitamin D assists the assimilation of vitamin A and maintains a healthy nervous system, normal heartbeat and efficient blood clotting.

It is mainly stored in the liver. In food, the vitamin is absorbed with fats through the intestines, and when produced by the sun, it is absorbed directly into the bloodstream. Typical deficiency symptoms include porous bones and teeth, leading to rickets, tooth decay, fatigue and arthritis, and one report links myopia (short-sightedness) to vitamin D deficiency. The vitamin is scarce in vegetables and its best natural sources include fish liver oil, sardines, herring, salmon, tuna and fortified milk. The recommended daily allowance is 400 i.u. for adults and children.

Caution: Prolonged daily doses above 1,600 i.u. can lead to over-accumulation and toxicity symptoms such as diarrhoea, nausea, excessive urination, calcification of arteries and kidney damage.

VITAMIN E

Vitamin E is a fat-soluble vitamin composed of a group of substances known as tocopherols, which are subdivided into alpha, beta, gamma, and so forth. Of these, alpha tocopherol is the most active. Vitamin E is available in both natural and synthetic forms, with the natural forms designated 'd' on supplement labels, as in d–alpha–tocopherol, and the synthetic forms designated 'dl', as in dl-alpha-tocopherol. The two forms are mirror images of one another, but only the natural 'd'–form is recognized by the body. 'Tocopherol' is derived from two Greek words meaning 'childbearing', since early studies of vitamin E were done with fertility problems.

Vitamin E is a most important lipid **antioxidant**. It binds oxygen and protects the fats in our bodies from the damaging effects of uncontrolled oxidation, peroxides and free radicals. These peroxides attack body cells, immune cells and cholesterol, reducing resistance and causing the degenerative diseases of ageing, such as cancer, heart attacks, strokes, arthritis, senility and diabetes. By binding oxygen, vitamin E alleviates some of the primary causes of death and helps to extend life-span. Vitamin E improves cell respiration (a boon to joggers), promotes fertility and sexual potency, is very effective in preventing the hot flushes of menopause and miscarriages, and protects the body from common pollutants such as ozone, radiation and toxic elements. The vitamin is used in the treatment of many conditions, including atherosclerosis, angina, hypertension, cancer, haemolytic anaemia, allergies, cataract, eczema, acne, premenstrual syndrome, skin ulcers, burns and digestive ulcers. A recent study has shown that a daily dose of 2,000 i.u. taken regularly can slow the deterioration resulting from Alzheimer's disease.

Vitamin E deficiency symptoms include fatigue and premature ageing, sterility and miscarriage, muscular dystrophy, haemolytic anaemia (which is not responsive to iron intake), circulatory disorders such as coronary thrombosis, varicose veins and thrombophlebitis, lameness due to poor circulation (claudication), kidney inflammation, degeneration of sex glands, and slow healing of wounds and burns. Among its best natural sources are raw wheat germ and wheat germ oil, vegetable oils, soybeans, whole grains, eggs and green leafy vegetables.

The recommended daily allowance of vitamin E is 15 i.u. for adults and 10.5 i.u. for children. However, for optimal protection, much higher doses are recommended. Vitamin E is available in potencies between 100 i.u. and 1,000 i.u. on its own, and it is also included in nutritional formulas. The most popular daily supplement is 400 i.u.

VITAMIN K

A fat-soluble vitamin, vitamin K tends to be a neglected nutrient because it is rarely deficient. It is known for its role in producing blood-clotting factors, such as prothrombin and, in this way, it contributes to the prevention of internal haemorrhaging and reduces excessive menstrual flow. It is also used to prevent haemorrhagic diseases in babies. In addition, vitamin K has recently been found to promote the building of healthy bones and to prevent osteoporosis.

Vitamin K occurs in three forms: K1 (phylloquinone), the natural vitamin K from plants; K2 (menaquinone), derived from intestinal bacteria; and K3 (menadione), which is the synthetic version of vitamin K available for those who cannot absorb it from food. To ensure adequate absorption and production of vitamin K in the body, cultured milk products such as yogurt and buttermilk, as well as vegetable oils, should be included in the daily diet. Antibiotics and overconsumption of sugar and sweets inhibit vitamin K absorption.

Deficiency symptoms include delayed blood-clotting of wounds, haemorrhages – such as nose bleeds, and a low level of blood platelets. Deficiencies of the vitamin are usually caused by a defect in metabolism, a malfunction of the liver, or by coeliac disease. Coeliac patients should emphasize vitamin K-rich foods in their diet and supplement with vitamins K, A, D and E, and also with calcium and the B-complex vitamins. The best natural sources of vitamin K include kale, green tea, alfalfa, spinach, broccoli, lettuce, cabbage, watercress, yogurt, egg yolk, fish liver oil and soybean oil. No official daily dosage has been established, but 300 mcg is generally considered adequate for an adult.

VITAMIN P SEE BIOFLAVONOIDS

W

WALNUTS *(Juglans Nigra)*

The tree, which probably originated in southern Europe, is now grown commercially in many parts of the world, especially in the US and China. Apart from the value of its timber, the tree is also noted for the culinary and medicinal properties of its nuts. Walnuts provide a good source of protein, iron and calcium and are used in traditional Chinese medicine to treat constipation and asthma. An infusion of walnut leaves can be used externally to treat eczema and improve the complexion. Walnut oil is used as a culinary oil, especially for salad dressings, and warmed walnut oil is a home remedy that is used externally for inflammation of the ear.

WATER

The most vital nutrient in our bodies, water makes up two-thirds of the body's mass and is involved in nearly every bodily process. Good, pure water is not only enlivening, but also nutritious. Although 'soft' water can be kinder to the skin when used externally, 'hard' water is nutritionally more beneficial to the body: it contains various minerals, especially calcium and magnesium, and is known to reduce the incidence of heart disease.

Unfortunately, contamination of tap water has become commonplace in recent years, due partly to the chemicals added at treatment plants and partly to contamination collected in the course of water distribution. Tap water is chlorinated and may cause allergies, diarrhoea or depression, as well as destroying friendly intestinal bacteria. It can also contain anti-corrosion chemicals added by some water boards, as well as environmental pollutants and industrial wastes. In addition, it may carry germs, algae, scale and rust particles which can contaminate the blood and lymph, overburdening the liver and kidneys with poisons, and lead to reduced energy and a lower resistance to disease. Since the purity and quality of water so greatly affects general health and well-being, it is no wonder that there is a growing public demand for higher quality water and that people are increasingly using bottled mineral waters, water filters and water purifiers.

As with any other nutrient, the body requires water in balanced amounts. Too much water, particularly after meals, will dilute digestive juices, weaken digestion and cause a sensation of coldness. Insufficient water intake will promote constipation, an accumulation of toxins, kidney damage, fatigue, apathy and dryness. Meat-based diets are known to increase thirst because they overload the body with uric acid and other by-products which need water for their dispersal. As a rule, vegetarians require less water than meat-eaters, since many fruits and vegetables contain over 90 per cent water. Grains and legumes, when cooked, contain about 80 per cent water, while the content of soups and teas is almost 100 per cent water. Optimal water requirements vary from person to person, and although thirst is the best indicator of need, it is not always reliable as it can sometimes be an indication of disease or disorder, such as diabetes. Each person must discover his or her own optimum requirement. However, experience shows that people tend to drink more water when good mineral water is available.

WATERCRESS *(NASTURTIUM OFFICINALIS)*

A perennial herb of the mustard family, it grows naturally in running water, especially the beds of streams, but is grown commercially in watercress beds or raised as a winter crop in greenhouses. Watercress is cultivated for its leaves, which are used mainly in salads, and are rich in vitamins and minerals, especially vitamins A, C, zinc and iron. The plant is also rich in potassium, calcium, phosphorus and iron, with good quantities of iodine, sodium and magnesium.

Although the healing powers of watercress have long been known, recent scientific studies have shown that it can inhibit the growth of some cancerous tumours. New research has revealed that fresh watercress contains high levels of PEITC (phenethyl isothiocyanate), which neutralizes a dangerous carcinogen in tobacco called NNK and one study indicated that the consumption of two ounces of fresh watercress three times a day for three days will help to protect smokers from lung cancer. For more lasting protection, this process can be repeated once a month.

A tea prepared from the leaves can strengthen digestion, increase urination, and cleanse the respiratory system by releasing phlegm and mucus and watercress is also recommended for the treatment of catarrh, anaemia, weak digestion and gout.

Caution: Excessive or prolonged use of watercress may cause kidney problems, and it should not be used in pregnancy. Since, nowadays, wild watercress grows mainly in polluted waters, it may contain various pollutants as well as the deadly liver fluke. Therefore, wild watercress is unsafe for gathering, and only watercress grown commercially in filtered, shallow, gravelled-bottom beds should be consumed.

WHEAT

Traditionally termed 'the staff of life', whole wheat is a highly nutritious grain and includes several varieties, such as bulgur and durum. Wheat starch contains anywhere between 6 and 20 per cent protein made up of eight amino acids. Wheat germ is a rich source of vitamin E, B vitamins and minerals such as zinc, iron, copper and iodine. The bran is rich in fibre and the amino acid lysine. Wheat encourages growth and can be used in conditions such as nervousness, insomnia and irritability. Being mildly astringent, wheat can be used for bed-wetting, diarrhoea and night sweats.

Sprouted wheat, particularly **wheat grass**, is an increasingly popular form of easily digestible wheat.

Standard white flour is made from the inner starchy part of the grain, with all the germ and bran removed. This results in a loss of up to 80 per cent of the essential nutrients in wheat. In addition, white flour may be bleached with chlorine dioxide, which destroys all the vitamin E. 'Enriched' flours make up for only a few of the missing nutrients, usually, vitamins B1, B2, B3 and iron.

Gluten, the elastic protein in wheat, is used as a popular source of vegetable protein in many dishes around the world. However, it can cause allergies and people with coeliac disease cannot digest it at all. The symptoms of coeliac disease, which is quite widespread, include diarrhoea, abdominal pain, flatulence, intestinal damage, weight loss and spasms. Coeliacs must not only avoid wheat, but all other gluten-containing cereals as well, and subsist on a gluten-free diet.

WHEAT GERM OIL

Produced from the life-giving part of the wheat kernel, wheat germ oil has been found to have many beneficial effects on the human body. It is the richest source of **vitamin E**, the great antioxidant and fertility vitamin. It is also the richest source of octacosanol, a type of waxy alcohol, the effects of which has a variety of effects on the body, including increased energy, endurance and strength, improved resistance to stress, alleviation of arthritis and improved heart function. In experiments done with the US Marines, wheat germ oil was found to relieve fatigue, dizziness, drowsiness and fear. In addition, animal studies have shown that wheat germ oil increases pregnancy rates and reduce miscarriages. Octacosanol has been found to have a remarkable therapeutic effect on muscular dystrophy and nerve–muscle disorders such as multiple sclerosis, epilepsy, cerebral palsy, encephalitis and myasthenia gravis. It has also been reported to regulate the blood clotting hormones, preventing blood clots and heart attacks.

The best wheat germ oil is cold pressed, fresh and packed in amber bottles. It is best kept in the refrigerator and taken in a dosage of a teaspoonful on empty stomach, one to three times daily.

Caution: Wheat germ oil contains significant amounts of oestrogen, the female sex hormone, and large doses over a prolonged period can cause testicular degeneration and loss of sex drive in men. For higher levels of supplementation, octacosanol tablets are safer and more beneficial.

WHEAT GRASS

Considered a 'living food', wheat grass is very rich in vitamin E, chlorophyll and many nutrients. It cleanses the blood, rejuvenates the body and increases resistance to disease. It is a tonic and helps to treat conditions such as fatigue, anaemia, toxaemia and cancerous growths.

Wheat grass juice is a powerful detoxifying agent. It helps to increase the enzyme level in the body cells, aiding the rejuvenation of the body and the digestion of nutrients. Wheat grass juice is best taken fresh on an empty stomach, starting off with an ounce a day, a daily dose which can gradually be increased up to four ounces. It is usually diluted with carrot or apple juice to make it more palatable.
More common in the US in larger health food stores where it can be bought as freshly squeezed juice.

WHEY

Whey is the water separated from milk during cheese-making after the milk has coagulated. It is considered highly nutritious and is the richest source of **lactose** (milk sugar). It is often added in dry form to processed foods, but is not suitable for people with lactose intolerance or for those allergic to milk.

Whey has recently found to contain certain proteins that can speed up the healing of wounds and ulcers. Initial studies were successfully conducted by Australian scientists who plan to use these whey ingredients in the form of dressings to accelerate wound repair. Other studies suggest that whey proteins may have anti-cancer and anti-microbial effects, as well as improving immune function.

Some products on the market already use whey. Estée

Lauder sells a moisturiser, called Nutritious, which uses whey protein to mimic a natural cellular messenger found in skin, which instructs it to produce more collagen. It's claimed, that it makes the skin stronger and more supple.

WILD YAM *(DIOSCOREA VILLOSA)* SEE YAM

WINE & BEER

The oldest beverage known to man, written records on the dietary and therapeutic uses of wine date back 4,000 years. Most of the today's wines come from a species of vine that originated in the Middle East, although in the US and Canada many of the varieties produced there have been crossbred with species native to North America.

Drunk in moderation, wine appears to be more than just an alcoholic or romantic drink. Red wine has been found to increase blood levels of **HDL** ('good' cholesterol) while decreasing **LDL** ('bad' cholesterol), and recent scientific research has indicated that two glasses of red wine a day can help to prevent blood clots, lower cholesterol, reduce the risk of heart attack and contribute to a longer life. Red wine is brewed from the full grapes, unlike white wine, and contains important antioxidant flavonoids such as **quercetin** and tannins, which account for its amazing benefits. It is these ingredients in red wine which have been put forward to explain the so called **French Paradox**, a phenomenon that has long baffled the scientific community.

Red wine is known to cause headaches or nasal congestions in some people and, although a controversial issue, it is suspected that these are allergic reactions to sulphites which are added to the wine to inhibit oxidation and microbial growth. Although most wine makers add sulphites, an increasing number are going 'organic', producing wine with no additives. (See also GRAPES; GRAPE SEEDS)

Beer is a relatively low alcoholic drink (4–8 per cent alcohol). The debate about its safety has both enthusiastic proponents and opponents. Moderate drinking seems to raise the level of the 'good' HDL cholesterol and prevent blockages in heart arteries in healthy people. However, a famous German study revealed that the alcohol did not benefit people with high cholesterol. Several other studies have suggested that light beer drinkers have less heart disease than heavy drinkers.

Heavy beer drinkers should remember that beer is high in purines, digestive byproducts that convert to uric acid, the buildup of which can bring on gout or worsen an existing one. Heavy beer drinking was found to increase the risk of rectal and lung cancer in men and breast cancer in women. It may also lead to cirrhosis of the liver, high blood pressure, varicose veins and piles, heart irregularities and foetal defects in pregnant women. Practicing moderation in beer drinking seems to be good advice.

WITCH HAZEL *(HAMAMELIS VIRGINIANA)*

A deciduous tree, which is native to North America, it was traditionally endowed with magical properties, hence its name. It is now grown in many other temperate regions of the world, including the British Isles.

The leaves of the witch hazel have an astringent, tonic and sedative effect. A decoction can be used for diarrhoea.

Extracts of witch hazel, which are available from most

herbalists, should be used only externally. As a skin lotion, the extract can be applied to bruises, insect bites and minor sunburns. A poultice is said to help in the treatment of haemorrhoids. The decoction can also be used as a mouth-wash and as a vaginal douche for vaginitis. Available from health food stores and herbalists.

WORMWOOD *(ARTEMISIA ABSINTHIUM)*

A silky perennial herb prevalent in arid roadside verges in Europe and North America, the leaves and flower tops of wormwood are used for several conditions. The leaves contain herbal bitters and santonin, which is effective against intestinal worms, and are used to prepare a bitter oil and also infusions. Wormwood is antiseptic and carminative, and can be used to stimulate the appetite and to treat indigestion. Wormwood oil is a cardiac stimulant and improves blood circulation.

Caution: Pure wormwood oil is poisonous and should only be used in correct dosages as indicated by a herbalist. Available from larger health food stores and herbalists.

Y

YAM, WILD YAM *(Dioscorea Villosa)*

Wild yam is a perennial vine with tuberous rootstock which is native to North America. Its roots yields an alkaloid which is a muscle relaxant, and it was used to treat abdominal cramps and bilious colics during the American Civil War. It can also be used to regularize menstruation and relieve menstrual cramps. One particular species of wild yam (D. vitata) has been found to contain up to 40 per cent diosgenin, a glycoside which can easily be converted to the hormone progesterone. (This hormone was previously produced from horse's urine.) In a study carried out over a four-year period, wild yam was found to be effective as an oral contraceptive, but without the side effects of the pill.

YARROW *(Achillea Millefolium)*

A herb which commonly grows wild along roadside verges, yarrow contains an essential oil and two acids, which together produce an astringent infusion that is aromatic and has a bitter taste. Traditionally, yarrow tea was used to induce sweating during a cold, and it is still recommended by herbalists for this purpose. An infusion of the plant can be used to alleviate digestive upsets, and arrest internal bleeding and heavy menstrual flow. Externally, it can be used as a soothing application for wounds, sore piles, and also as a mouthwash in cases of gum inflammation and as a hair tonic.

Available from herbalists.

Caution: Yarrow can cause dermatitis in some people.

YEAST SEE BREWER'S YEAST

YOGURT

Increasingly publicized as a health food, yogurt has been used for centuries by many of the long-living ethnic societies. Now rediscovered as a **probiotic** food, yogurt is simply milk that has been fermented by several strains of bacteria, such as **Lactobacillus acidophilus** and **Bifidobacteria bifidum**. The bacteria curdle the milk by converting the milk sugar to lactic acid. One of the main nutritional benefits of yogurt is to reinforce the intestines with additional 'friendly' bacteria, promoting the growth of intestinal flora. The bacteria of the intestinal flora aid digestion and absorption of food, produce B vitamins, prevent the growth of pathogenic bacteria (such as candida) which cause diseases, and inhibit internal decay; they also promote a healthy intestinal acidity. In this respect, yogurt is especially beneficial to people on antibiotics, and for those who have a sweet tooth or who drink chlorinated water, all of which deplete friendly bacteria. Yogurt also helps to synthesize vitamin K, preventing internal haemorrhages, and it lowers cholesterol levels and reduces the risk of cancer, especially colon cancer.

However, apart from these benefits, yogurt is also a highly nutritious food. It is a good source of quality protein, vitamins and minerals: it contains vitamins A, B complex, E and D, and is an excellent source of easily absorbed calcium, potassium and phosphorus, and contains only a moderate amount of sodium. Yogurt is also easily digestible – in fact, most of its protein is digested within an hour. It is also a highly valuable food for the treatment of gastroenteritis, colitis, constipation, bilious disorders, flatulence, bad breath, high cholesterol, migraine and nervous fatigue. In addition, yogurt can often be taken by people who cannot use other forms of milk due to lactose intolerance.

YOHIMBE *(PAUSINYSTALIA JOHIMBE)*

In recent years, yohimbe capsules have swept health food stores in the US as a potent aphrodisiac. The bark of the yohimbe plant, which is a native of South America, contains yohimbine, and this was approved by the US FDA (Food and Drug Administration) for the treatment of erectile dysfunction. Although yohimbine can increase sex drive, its primary action is to increase blood flow to the erectile tissue. It has no effect, however, on testosterone levels. When used on its own, yohimbe can help about a third of cases. However, its side effects, which in some people can include depression, anxiety, hallucinations, headaches, hypertension, dizziness or skin flushing, make it difficult to use. Both yohimbe and yohimbine are therefore best used under medical supervision.

Z

ZINC

An essential trace element, zinc is found in every cell of the body and performs numerous useful functions. It is a component of some 200 **enzymes** and is involved in more enzymatic reactions than any other mineral. It is a constituent of **insulin**, growth hormones and sex hormones, and is richly contained in human sperm. It takes part in carbohydrate metabolism, the breakdown of **alcohol** and the synthesis of **nucleic acids**. Together with **vitamins A, B6** and **B12**, zinc is necessary for proper growth. It also aids the excretion of toxic cadmium found in cigarette smoke (which causes hypertension), and neutralizes the bad effects of excess copper (a cause of arthritis). Zinc is crucial for the maturation of the sex glands and for their function, particularly the prostate. It prevents enlargement of the prostate, which can block urine flow and is a common source of distress for many men over 45.

Together with vitamin B6, zinc inhibits histamine production and is therefore helpful in treating allergies. It soothes nerves and depression and is used in the treatment of Alzheimer's disease and some types of schizophrenia. Zinc can also speed up the healing of wounds and is used to cure ulcers resulting from cortisone treatment. Due to its presence in insulin, zinc increases the insulin effect and is therefore helpful in the treatment of diabetes. It has also been found to boost natural immunity against disease and is well-known for its ability to promote skin health and alleviate psoriasis. For this reason, it is sometimes used as an ingredient in skin creams.

The symptoms of zinc deficiency are many and varied. They include swollen prostate, sterility, impotence and delayed sexual maturation in children, stunted growth, menstrual irregularities, susceptibility to infections and poor wound healing, joint pains, atherosclerosis and poor circulation, slow learning and mental retardation, loss of sense of taste and smell, allergies, acne, stretch marks in pregnant women, white spots in nails, offensive perspiration, and susceptibility to diabetes.

Zinc is depleted by alcohol and smoking, and profuse sweating can cause a loss of up to 3 mg a day. Among the best natural sources of the mineral are raw oysters, clams, meat, fish, raw wheat germ, brewer's yeast, mushrooms, pumpkin seeds, egg yolks, legumes. The recommended daily allowance is 15 mg for adults and 10 mg for children. Requirements increase during pregnancy or lactation. Zinc supplements in strengths of up to 40 mg are available in health food stores.

Helpful addresses for general herbal advice

U.K.

The British Herbal Medicine Association (BHMA)
   Sun House, Church Street, Stroud, Gloucestershire GL5 1JL
The National Institute of Medical Herbalists
   9 Palace Gate, Exeter, Devon EX1 1JA
The Herb Society
   77 Great Peter Street, London SW1
General Council and Register of Consultant Herbalists, Grosvenor
   House, 40 Sca Way, Middleton-on-Sea, W. Sussex, PO22 7SA

U.S.A.

The American Botanical Council, P.O. Box 201660, Austin, Texas 78720
The Herb Research Foundation, 1007 Pearl Street, Suite 200, Boulder
   Colorado 80302
American Herb Association, P.O.B. 353, Rescue, CA 95672
California School of Herbal Studies, P.O.B. 39, Forestville, CA 95436.

Australia

National Herbalist Association of Australia, 27 Leith Street, Coorparoo,
   Queensland 4151

Herbal Suppliers

U.K.

Potters Herbal Suppliers, Leyland Mill Lane, Wigan, Lancashire WN1 2SB
   Tel: 0942 34761
Culpepper Ltd, 21 Bruton Street, Berkeley Square, London W1X 7OA
Neal's Yard Apothecary, 2 Neal's Yard, Covent Garden, London WC2
   Tel: 0171 379 7222
A. Nelson & Co. Ltd, Heritage House, 21 Inner Park Road, Wimbeldon,
   London SW19 6ED

U.S.A.

Nature's Herbs, 113 North Industrial Park Drive, Orem, Utah 84057
Tel: 801 225 4443
Nature's Way, P.O. Box 4000, Springville, Utah 84883
Tel: 800-9-NATURE
eclectic Institute, 11231 S.E. Market Street, Portland, Oregon 97216
Tel: 800-332-HERB
Wakunaga, 23501 Madero, Mission Viejo, California 92691
Tel: 800-544-5800
Acta Health Products, 1979 East Locust Street, Pasadena, California 91107
Four Seasons Herb Company, 17 Buccaneer Street, Marinal Del Rey,
California 90292 (Specializes in oriental herbs)
Bio-Botanica, Inc., 75 Commerce Drive, Hauppauge, New York 11788
Tel: 516 231 5522
Earthrise Company, P.O. Box 1196, San Rafael, California 94915
Tel: 415 485 0521
Threshold, 23 Janesway, Scotts Valley, California 95066
Tel: 408 438 1144
Excel, 3280 West Hacienda, Las Vegas, Nevada 89041
Tel: 702 795 7464
Yerba Prima, P.O. Box 5009, Berkeley, California 94705
Tel: 415 632 7477

Canada

Trophic Canada Ltd. 260 Okanagan Avenue East, Penticton, BC V2A357
Tel: 604 492 8820
Flora Distributors Ltd. 7400 Fraser Park Drive, Burnaby, BC VSJ5B9
Tel: 604 438 1133
Swiss Herbal Remedies, 181 Don Park Road, Markham, Ontario L3RIC2
Tel: 416 475 6345
Quest, 1781 West 75th Avenue, Vancouver, BC V6P6P2
Tel: 604 261 0611
The Herb Works, PO Box 450, Fergus, Ontario N1M1N8
Tel: 519 824 4280
Vita Health, 150 Beghin Avenue, Winnipeg, MBR1J3W2
Tel: 204 661 8386
Bio-Force, 4001 Cote Verth, Montreal, PQ H4R1R5
Tel: 514 335 9393

INDEX